High Vibration Nutrition

A Simple Guide to a Holistic Plant-based Lifestyle

BaNAuset KaNSekhmet, BSN, RN

High Vibration Nutrition:

A Simple Holistic Guide to a Plant-based Lifestyle

ISBN: 978-1-63625-777-8

Copyright © 2021

Author: BaNAuset KaNSekhmet

Publisher: Kemetic Wellness Sacred Healing Center

www.kemeticwellness.com

Dedication

This book is dedicated to all the keepers of African Natural Medicine who reminded me that our healing is in our culture. To my teachers, both direct and indirect, who guided me from death to resurrection. To my future children, may this work contribute to a life of wellness, that we may heal our family seven generations past and seven generations future. To the children of the African diaspora, may this work assist in leading you back to your birth rite of mind, body and spiritual wellness.

Table of Contents

PREFACE

I was born in the Bronx, NY on September 4th, 1985, to two Jamaican parents— Iris M. Thompson and James Samuel Green. From an early age, I displayed a natural intelligence and talents for the healing and performing arts. I began school at age 3 in Bronx Baptist Church's preschool. At age 5 I entered Public School 85 at the kindergarten level. By then, I was already an avid reader and loved writing. At age 8, I entered P.S. 85's gifted performing arts program. There I was able to practice and cultivate my music, theater and writing skills. The program was most known for its yearly Christmas plays, which the entire school anticipated. Although I was quite shy about performing on stage, I truly loved the creativity involved in production. I was quite determined not to let my stage freight keep me from acting on stage with my classmates.

From elementary school, I moved on to PACE Academy, another gifted program at Middle School 118. There I excelled in languages such as English, Latin, and Spanish and was also awarded for my talents in creative design. At age 14, I enrolled in DeWitt Clinton High School's Medical Science Honor (MACY) Program.

It was in high school that I started to become more aware of the troubles facing my community. Gang violence, drug addiction, poverty, parental abandonment and teenage pregnancy were just a few of the ills I witnessed in my Bronx neighborhood. Yet, I envisioned myself being a part of the solution. In my Sophomore year of high school, I joined my school's Helping Hands Club, a volunteer organization where I got my start in coordinating community service activities. As a volunteer, I visited the elderly at St. Patrick's nursing home to keep them company. During my junior and senior years of high school, I would spend my Saturdays volunteering at P.O.T.S (Part of the Solution) Soup Kitchen. I also began volunteering for ASPIRA, another community service organization in the Bronx. One of my most memorable projects with ASPIRA was the beautification of a school playground in the Bronx.

When it was time to prepare for college, it was my father who convinced me to take up nursing, and it was an easy sell. After high school, I enrolled at Adelphi University's School of Nursing. There I quickly naturally gravitated towards their community service club C.A.L.I.B.E.R. - Cause to Achieve Leadership Intelligence Brotherhood Excellence and Respect. C.A.L.I.B.E.R. is a chapter of Circle K International- the largest collegiate community service organization worldwide. There I played a key role in planning events and fundraising for numerous causes, including Ronald McDonald House of Long Island, Operation Christmas Child, the March of Dimes and the Caroline Wambui Mungai Foundation.

I earned a Bachelor of Science degree in Nursing from Adelphi University and obtained New York State licensure as a Registered Professional Nurse in 2008.

I began my nursing career at Harlem Hospital Center's Inpatient Pediatric Unit. As the youngest nurse on my unit, I had to adapt quickly. Other nurses soon observed that I had a knack for dealing with the "difficult patients"— the "angry," "crazy" ones who would curse the staff out. As charge nurse, I consistently cared for these patients. I practiced nursing from a place of empathy, which allowed me to see what people needed without them having to say it. I quickly gained a reputation, among my patients and medical team, for running a smooth unit and handling patients with kindness and ease. After four years of clinical experience, I became the first Certified Pediatric Nurse in my unit.

Through my work as a nurse, I heard the frustrations of the Black community, who needed natural, cultural care and spiritual healing. I resigned from my position at Harlem Hospital in 2014, hoping to find a more therapeutic healthcare setting aligned with my vision of wellness. I was confused about why there was little to no emphasis on nutrition and even more disheartened to learn that none of the health institutions I subsequently worked for had any interest in the patients' healing. After moving from one institution to the next, I quickly learned that they were all operating under the same sick-care system. As my eyes began to open to these realities, I became more passionate about natural living as a means to treat and prevent illness.

In my quest to figure out how to use my medical training to help my community through natural methods, I was divinely guided to the teachings of ancient Kemet. I was initiated into the Kemetic tradition by Grand Master and Kemetic High Priest, Mfundishi Jhutyms. I began studying the ancient Kemetic language, healing arts and spiritual sciences. Through these teachings, I learned that the healing of African people is in embracing and returning to African culture.

One of my most significant transformations was my name. In the Kemetic tradition, your name is the utterance of your energy. It connects you to a land mass, a history, and a culture. Every time your name is spoken it is an affirmation of your purpose. From this African-centered paradigm I changed my birth name, Latasha Green, to my cultural name, BaNAuset KaNSekhmet.

As I fully immersed myself in the ancient Kemetic healing practices, I was attuned to RaSekhi Kemetic Reiki by Master Teacher MutShat Shemsut-Gianprem. I then began to study womb health and wisdom under the guidance of Supreme Medicine Woman, Queen Afua. I completed Queen Afua's Sacred Woman Rites of Passage and was among the first graduating class of Womb Yoga Dance Practitioners at the Queen Afua Wellness University. I further studied African Holistic Health under Dr. Akua Gray and became Certified as a Natural Health and Wellness Consultant.

These teachings led to the birth of Kemetic Wellness Sacred Healing Center. The African Holistic Health wisdom that transformed my life is infused into the foundation of Kemetic Wellness Sacred Healing Center, a non-profit community organization dedicated to providing African holistic health services, education and products. I opened the doors to my wellness center in Yonkers, NY, in May 2018. It is the mission of Kemetic Wellness Sacred Healing Center to use these ancient African healing tools and techniques to help create a healthy, prosperous community.

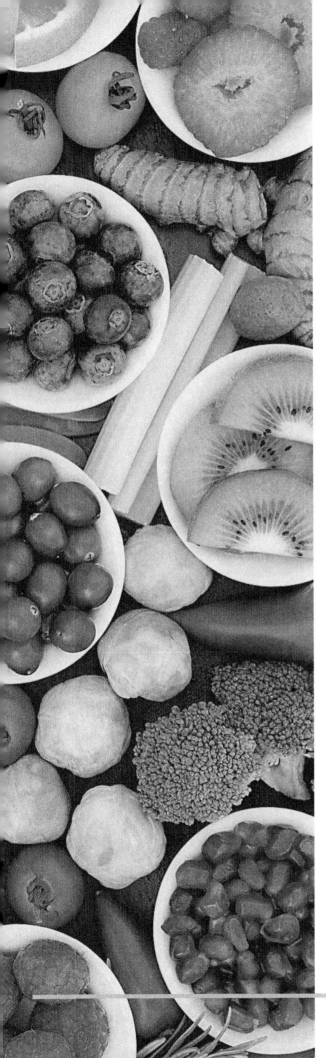

Introduction:
High Vibration Nutrition
High Vibration Life

Food is life! It fuels our bodies with the nutrients needed to carry out all of the body's necessary functions. It connects us culturally and socially. We take on the energy of the foods we consume, which can either heighten or lower our energetic frequency. Low-frequency nutrition negatively affects our mental, emotional and physical health. When our bodies are properly nourished, our cells vibrate at a higher frequency, and we maximize our ability to function at our highest capacity.

As a living being, you can only truly refuel with living things. Our cells need water, sunlight and minerals such as calcium and phosphorus to facilitate proper organ functioning. When our bodies are well-nourished with these minerals our cells can function at an optimal level, raising our vibrational frequency. Natural, organic, live-foods are nutrient-rich, and can therefore provide proper nourishment for the body.

Artificial, processed and denatured foods have no life and therefore cannot give us life. Instead, they strip nutrients from the body and, over time, create an internal environment that is acidic and prone to disease. A diet that is rich in high vibration, natural foods creates an optimal internal environment for the body where disease cannot exist. I encourage you to use this simple nutritional guide in transitioning from a nutrient-deficient, standard Western Diet to a high vibration, plant-based diet for a life of optimal wellness.

Vibrational Frequency And Nutrition

Frequency is the rate at which a vibration occurs per unit of time, creating a specific energetic field. Frequency is measured in units of Hz (hertz), which is equal to one occurrence of a repeating event per second. Commonly used multiples are kHz (kilohertz, 103 Hz), MHz (megahertz, 106 Hz), GHz (gigahertz, 109 Hz) and THz (terahertz, 1012 Hz).

Everything that exists is vibrating on a particular frequency. The ancient Africans of Kemet called this internal vital energy *sekhem,* also known as *moyo* in Swahili, *chi* in Chinese and *qi* in Japanese. As energetic beings, everything we come into contact with can either raise or lower our vibrational frequency. The state of your physical body, emotions and thoughts influence your frequency. Devitalized foods, pollution, traumatic events, arguments, negative self-talk, anger, worry and stress all negatively alter your energetic frequency. When the frequency drops, the immune system is compromised. Substances with a high frequency create an energetic environment that destroys diseases that vibrate on a lower frequency.

One of the first biofrequency monitors was built by Dr. Royal Raymond Rife in the late 1920s. Dr. Raymond found that certain frequencies can prevent disease development and that others would even destroy it. The application of using certain frequencies to heal the body had already been suggested by the American inventor Nikola Tesla (1856 – 1943), who pioneered Western electrical technology. According to Tesla: "If you could eliminate certain outside frequencies that interfered with our bodies, we would have greater resistance toward disease." In 1992, researcher Bruce Tainio built a frequency monitor and discovered that a healthy human body vibrates on a frequency of 62-78 MHz.

Disease begins at a biofrequency of 57-60 MHz, where the body becomes susceptible to colds and flu. Candida overgrowth starts at a frequency of 55 MHz. At 52 MHz, the body becomes receptive to Epstein Barr Virus. Cancer develops at a vibrational frequency of 42 MHz, and death is imminent at 25 MHz or lower.

Nature offers every healing substance necessary to raise our *sekhem.* Essential oils resonate at the highest biofrequencies known to mankind, beginning at 52 MHz and going up to 320 MHz. Rose oil has the highest frequency of all essential oils at 320 MHz. Other foods within this range include chlorophyll, phytoplankton and wheatgrass. Phytoplankton alone provides the Earth with 50-85% of its oxygen.

Fresh foods from the tree, which are generally consumed raw, range between 20-27 MHz because of their high mineral content. This includes apples, avocado, bananas, blueberries, cherries, coconut, dates, lychee, melons, raspberries, pineapple, and mango. The frequency of these foods can be higher if grown organically and eaten freshly picked. Superfoods grown organically, such as raw nuts and seeds, raw chocolate, fresh herbs of all kinds, lemons, limes, Goji berries, mangosteen, soursop, and sea vegetables (like chlorella, dulse, Irish moss, kelp, and spirulina) have even higher frequencies. Dried foods and herbs range slightly lower between 12-22 MHz. Processed foods, canned foods, animal discharge (dairy, eggs, butter, etc.) and dead flesh (hot dogs, burgers, meat, shrimp, lobster, etc.) resonate at 0 MHz.

The consumption of high vibrational foods has the ability to increase your own natural electromagnetic vibrations and restore MAAT (balance and order) to your electric fields to produce and maintain wellness. Lower vibrational foods rob your body of energy because your body's energy is used to process and digest these foods, which yield absolutely nothing in return. Over time, consistent consumption of low vibrational foods depletes your electromagnetic field leaving you prone to illness, and eventually death.

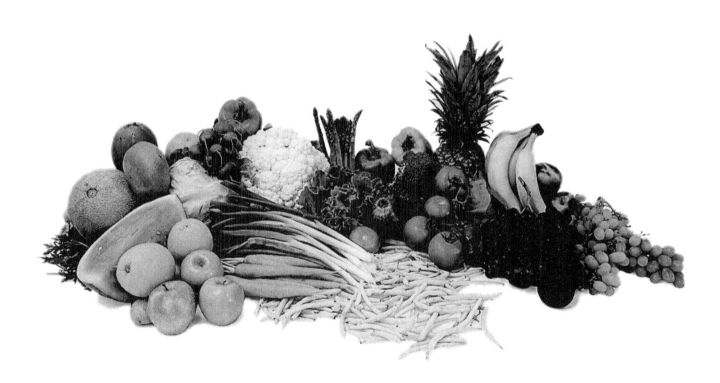

High Vibration Foods: Macronutrients

High quality, nutrition-packed, electric, life-giving foods.

Organic and locally grown produce.

Increase vitality, mood and organ function.

Allow the body to heal from dis-ease.

Staple foods.

Carbohydrates

Function: provide the body with energy

70% of daily caloric intake

4 calories per gram

Fresh fruit: cleanses, detoxifies, contains high mineral content

- Apple, Apricot, Banana, Blueberry, Cactus Fruit, Cherries, Coconut, Fig, Grapes, Grapefruit, Guineps, Guava, Jackfruit, June Plum, Lemon, Lychee, Mangosteen, Mango, Naseberry (Sapodilla), Orange, Papaya, Passion Fruit, Peach, Pear, Persimmon, Pineapple, Plum, Plantains, Pomegranate, Rambutan, Raspberry, Star Apple, Strawberry, Starfruit, Soursop, Sweetsop, Tamarind, Tangerine, Watermelon.

- Fruits eaten as vegetables: Ackee, Avocado, Green Banana, Breadfruit, Tomato.

Vegetables: strengthen, repair and heal

- Beet, Bell Pepper, Broccoli, Brussels Sprouts, Cabbage, Callaloo, Cauliflower, Celery, Chayote, Chives, Cucumber, Eggplant, Leeks, Okra, Onions, Rhubarb, Scallion, Sprouts, Tomatillo, Wheatgrass, Zucchini.

- Leafy Greens: Arugula, Beet Greens, Butterhead Lettuce, Dandelion Greens, Collard Greens, Endives, Spinach, Kale, Mustard Greens, Romaine Lettuce, Swiss Chard, Turnip Greens, Watercress.

- Ground provisions (root vegetables): Arrowroot, Butternut Squash, Daikon, Carrot, Beet, Dasheen Root, Eddos, Burdock, Parsnips, Potato, Pumpkin, Radishes, Squash, Sweet Potato, Rutabaga, Yam, Taro, Turnips.

- Organic whole grains: Amaranth, Barley, Basmati Rice, Black Rice, Brown Rice, Buckwheat, Bulgar, Corn, Cornmeal, Couscous, Fonio, Jasmine Rice, Kamut, Millet, Oat, Quinoa, Rye, Spelt, Semolina, Teff, Wild Rice, Wheatgerm.

- Whole-grain bread: Rye, Semolina, Spelt, Sunflower Seed Bread, Injera.

- Whole-grain pasta: Spelt, Quinoa, Brown Rice, Whole Wheat, Sprouted-Grain, Buckwheat noodles.

Proteins

Function: build and repair tissues, make enzymes, hormones and other body chemicals

15% of daily caloric intake

4 calories per gram

- Legumes: Black Beans, Black-eyed Peas, Cannelloni beans, Chickpeas, Kidney Beans, Lentils, Lima Beans, Navy Beans, Pinto Beans, Alfalfa Sprouts, Fava beans, Mung Bean Sprouts, String Beans, Snow Peas, Sugar Snap Peas.

- Mushrooms: Button, Chanterelles, Cremini, Enoki, King Trumpet, Morels, Oyster, Porcini, Portabello, Reishi, Shitake.

- Nuts and Seeds: Almonds, Cashews, Chia Seeds, Hazelnut, Hemp Seeds, Flax Seeds, Macadamias, Peanuts, Pine Nuts, Pistachios, Poppy Seeds, Pumpkin Seeds, Sesame Seeds, Sunflower Seeds, Walnuts.

- High Protein Greens: Asparagus, Artichokes, Arugula, Broccoli, Brussels Sprouts, Cauliflower, Corn, Beet Greens, Broccoli Raab, Okra, Potato, Turnip Greens

- Sea Vegetables: Bladderwrack, Chlorella, Dulse, Irish Moss, Kelp, Kombu, Nori, Sea Lettuce, Seaweed, Spirulina.

- Seitan: a meat substitute made from wheat gluten, which can be flavored or cooked in vegan or vegetarian dishes.

Fats

Function: to support cell growth, protect organs, maintain normal body temperature, and help the body to absorb nutrients

15% of daily caloric intake

9 calories per gram

- Fatty fruits such as Avocado, Coconut and Olives

- Oils best for cooking: Grapeseed Oil, Avocado Oil, Peanut Oil, Palm Oil

- Oils best for dressings and flavorings: Extra Virgin Olive Oil, Flaxseed, Sunflower, Sesame Oils, unrefined Coconut Oil

- Nuts and Seeds: Almonds, Brazil Nuts, Cashews, Chia Seeds, Hazelnuts, Hemp Seeds, Flax Seeds, Macadamias, Peanuts, Pecans, Pine Nuts, Pistachios, Poppy Seeds, Pumpkin Seeds, Sesame Seeds, Sunflower Seeds, Walnuts

- Nut butter: Almond Butter, Cashew Butter, Peanut Butter

- Vegan butter spread

- Vegan mayonnaise

- Vegan cheese: Almond Cheese, Cashew Cheese

Liquids

Daily water intake: Drink half your body weight (by the pound) in ounces

(Ex: a 140 lb. woman should consume 70 oz or 8.75 cups of water daily)

- Fresh vegetable and fruit juices and smoothies

- Herbal teas

- Plant-based milk: almond milk, coconut milk, hazelnut milk, hemp milk, oat milk, rice milk

- Purified, distilled or spring water

- Vegetable soups

- Infused water

Sweets

Use Sparingly

- Dried Fruit: Apple, Banana, Coconut, Cranberry, Dates, Kiwi, Goji Berries, Mango, Pineapple, Prunes, Raisins.

- Sweeteners: Agave, Blackstrap Molasses, Honey, Grade B Maple Syrup, Stevia Leaf, Unrefined Cane Sugar, Coconut Sugar, Coconut Condensed Milk.

Spices & condiments

Use Sparingly

- Apple cider vinegar

- Liquid aminos

- Hummus

- Nutritional yeast

- Organic Ketchup

- Siracha

- Tahini

- Tamari

- Tamarind

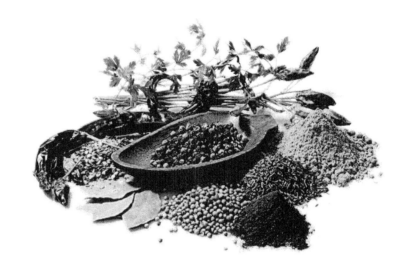

Herbs

- Alfalfa (asthma)

- Basil (anti-inflammatory)

- Cayenne Pepper (circulation)

- Cascara Sagrada (laxative)

- Celery (balance pH)

- Cerasee (blood cleanser)

- Chamomile (relaxation)

- Cinnamon (regulates blood sugar)

- Citrus Peel (improve digestion)

- Cloves (antiseptic, anesthetic)

- Coriander (diarrhea, gas)

- Cumin (anti-congestive, respiratory issues)

- Curry (immune booster, cancer protection)

- Dandelion (blood tonic)

- Dill (supports urinary system)

- Fennel (gas, heartburn, bloating)

- Fenugreek (blood sugar control, lowers cholesterol)

- Garlic (antibiotic)

- Ginger (increases circulation, anti-inflammatory)

- Goldenseal (antibiotic)

- Hibiscus (lowers BP and cholesterol)
- Kelp (source of iodine)
- Lemongrass (fever)
- Maca root (hormone balance)
- Moringa (nutrient-dense superfood)
- Neem (skin ailments)
- Nutmeg (indigestion)
- Onion (anti-cancer)
- Oregano (respiratory system)
- Paprika (pain relief)
- Parsley (breath freshener)
- Peppermint (aids digestion, cooling effect)
- Red Raspberry Leaf (menstrual irregularities)
- Sage (improves cognitive function)
- Sea Salt (source of iodine)
- Sorel (effective against high blood pressure and uterine fibroids)
- Spearmint (nausea relief)
- Thyme (parasites)
- Turmeric (pain, anti-inflammatory)
- Valerian (insomnia)

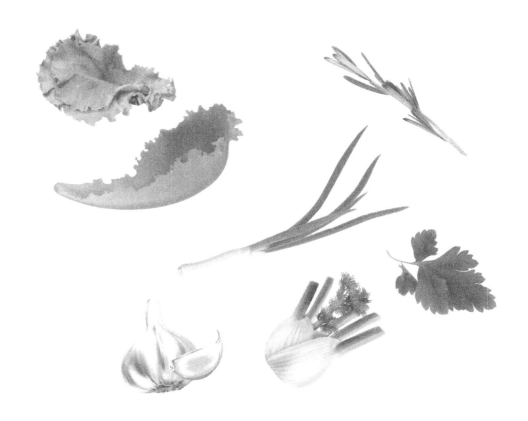

High Vibration Foods: Micronutrients

Essential Vitamins, Minerals and Amino Acids

Micronutrients are essential elements required by the human body to orchestrate a range of physiological functions for maintaining health and life. Almost 99% of the human body mass is made up of six elements: oxygen, carbon, hydrogen, nitrogen, calcium, and phosphorus. Only about 0.85% is composed of another five elements: potassium, sulfur, sodium, chlorine, and magnesium. All 11 are necessary for life. The human body mass contains at least detectable traces of 60 chemical elements. About 29 of these elements play an active, positive role in life and health in humans.

Minerals are made up of organic elements. Some minerals are made up of just one element, although most are compounds. Vitamins and minerals are considered essential nutrients because they act in synergy, performing countless roles in the body. They build up bones, muscles, regulate proper organ functioning, heal wounds and boost your immune system. They convert food into energy and repair cellular damage.

Amino acids are organic compounds composed of nitrogen, carbon, hydrogen, oxygen, along with a variable side chain group. These compounds combine to form proteins. Amino acids are the necessary building blocks in the formation of proteins. There are over 20 amino acids necessary for proper growth and organ function, although only 9 are classified as essential. Essential amino acids are vital to human life and must be obtained from food, as they cannot be synthesized in the body. Conditionally essential amino acids can be synthesized in the body, but in certain circumstances, you need to get them from food. Our bodies produce nonessential amino acids, even if we don't get them from food.

Listed below are some nutrients that are essential for proper organ functioning, metabolism and good health.

Nutrients/ Recommended Daily Allowance	Function	Deficiency Symptoms	Toxicity Symptoms	Natural Food Sources
		Fat-Soluble Vitamins		
Vitamin A • 900 mcg (men) 700 mcg (women) • Fat-soluble Vitamin	Eyesight, bone growth, reproduction, appetite and test, immune system regulation.	Night-blindness, dry skin, macular degeneration, nerve damage.	Nausea, vomiting, headaches, insomnia, dry skin, joint pain, constipation.	Asparagus, Carrots, Green Leafy Vegetables, Pumpkin, Spinach, Turnip Greens, Yams, Yellow Fruits. Herbs: Alfalfa, Comfrey, Dandelion, Eyebright, Paprika, Parsley, Peppermint Raspberry Leaves, Watercress.
Vitamin D • 400-800 IU • Fat soluble • Is both a vitamin and a hormone	Necessary for glandular function, especially thyroid. Aids absorption and utilization of minerals. Strengthens bones teeth, muscles, heart. Essential for normal blood clotting and regulates heart beat.	Bone deformities, cancer, delayed tooth development in children, hypocalcemia, hypoglycemia, osteoarthritis, osteomalacia, osteoporosis, rickets, weak muscles.	Nausea, vomiting, headaches, constipation, diarrhea, fatigue, loss of appetite, excessive thirst and urination, proteinuria, liver and kidney damage.	Dandelion greens, Lettuce, Mushrooms, Oatmeal, Sweet Potatoes, Yams. Sun exposure. Herbs: Alfalfa, Horsetail, Parsley, Nettle, Watercress.

Vitamin E • 30-1,200 IU • Fat soluble vitamin	Essential for the health of lungs, skin, blood, heart, veins and arteries. Antioxidant. Promotes healthy tissues, healing of sores, good circulation, stabilizes energy, and lowers blood pressure. Good for stamina, protects prostate, blood thinner, relaxes muscles and reduces wound scarring.	Anemia, cataracts, diarrhea, flatulence, edema, eye disorders, increased triglycerides, keloids, nausea, PMS, prolonged clotting time, prostate problems, sterility, impotency, menopause, all infections and disease.	Generally considered nontoxic, but upset stomach, dizziness, and diarrhea can occur.	Corn, Green Leafy Vegetables, Nuts, Oatmeal, Rice, Safflower, Spinach, Sprouted Seeds, Sunflower seeds, Sweet potatoes, Vegetable and Nut Oils, Wheat germ, Whole grains, Yams. Herbs: Alfalfa, Bladderwrack, Dandelion, Dong Quai, Kelp, Rosehip, Spirulina, Watercress.
Vitamin K • 80-125 mg • Fat soluble vitamin	Vital for making prothrombin that makes blood clot (thicken), liver, bone formation and repair, nervous system and energy. helps to stop heavy menstruation and long bleeding periods.	Easy bruising or bleeding, celiac disease, cystic fibrosis, intestinal or binary tract (liver, gallbladder and bile ducts) disorder, black tar-like stools, small blood clots under the nails.	Generally nontoxic, but a type of neonatal jaundice may occur in premature infants; elevated levels of vitamin K can interfere with the effects of anticoagulants.	Asparagus, Broccoli, Brussels Sprouts, Cabbage, Cauliflower, Green Leafy Vegetables, Oatmeal, Rye, Soybeans, Wheat. Herbs: Alfalfa, Kelp, Nettle, Oatstraw, Plantain, Shepherd's Purse.

Coenzyme Q10 • 90-200 mg daily • Fat-soluble vitamin-like substance	Improves oxygenation in tissue and circulation. Boosts immunity. Combats, asthma, allergies, respiratory disease. Prevents and treats cardiac disease. An antioxidant. Reduces tumors. Aids the stomach lining and duodenum.	Extreme fatigue and muscle weakness, poor muscle tone, dystonia. Problems with coordination and balance. Brain dysfunction, seizures and intellectual disabilities. Eye and ear problems.	Generally nontoxic.	Cauliflower, Broccoli, Legumes, Nuts, Oranges, Pistachios, Seeds, Spinach, Sesame Seeds, Strawberries.
Water Soluble Vitamins				
Vitamin B1 *Thiamine* • 25-300 mg • Water-soluble Vitamin	Nervous system, digestion, muscles, heart, alcohol-damaged nerve tissue, circulation, brain function.	Appetite and weight loss, nausea, vomiting, fatigue, nervous system problems, muscle weakness, edema, enlarged heart.	Generally nontoxic.	Asparagus, Beans, Broccoli, Brown Rice, Brussels sprouts, Oranges, Raisins, Raw Peanuts, Rice Bran, Peas, Plums, Wheat Germ. Herbs: Alfalfa, Burdock Roots, Dandelion, Eyebright, Fennel, Parsley.

Vitamin B2 *Riboflavin* • 25-300 mg • Water-soluble Vitamin	Growth, skin, hair, nails, eyesight, digestion of fat, protein and carbohydrates	Cracks and sores on tongue and corners of mouth, red eyes, skin lesions, dizziness, hair loss, sleep loss, sensitivity to light, poor digestion, anemia.	Generally nontoxic.	Almonds, Asparagus, Avocado, Brewer's Yeast, Broccoli, Currants, Green Leafy Vegetables, Mushrooms, Spinach, Sunflower seeds, Whole grains. Herbs: Alfalfa, Burdock, Chickweed, Garlic, Kelp, Parsley.
Vitamin B3 *Nicotinic acid (niacin)* • Water-soluble Vitamin • 25-300 mg	Nervous system, skin, circulation, digestion, sex hormones, mental acuity, memory, lowers cholesterol	Canker sores, diarrhea, dizziness, fatigue, halitosis, headaches, indigestion, insomnia, mental illness, dermatitis, hypoglycemia.	**Mild:** Nausea, vomiting, abdominal cramps, diarrhea, flushing. **Severe:** Liver damage, irregular heartbeat, rash to large portions of the body, gouty arthritis.	Brewer's Yeast, Broccoli, Carrots, Dandelion Greens, Dates, Green Leafy Vegetables, Peanuts, Potatoes, Tomatoes, Whole Wheat, Sunflower Seeds, Brown Rice, Nuts. Herbs: Alfalfa, Burdock, Cayenne, Garlic, Fenugreek, Nettle, Red Raspberry, Yellow Dock.
Vitamin B5 *Pantothenic acid* • 25-500 mg • Water-soluble vitamin	Adrenal glands and hormones, cortisone pro-duction and re-laxation aids in the metabolism of macro nutri-ents for energy, helps to make neurotransmit-ters.	Alleries, asthma, hair loss, fatigue, mental problems, skin disease, burning feet, headaches, dizziness, hypoglycemia, low blood pressure.	Generally nontoxic.	Bran, Brewer's Yeast, Fresh Vegetables, Legumes, Mushrooms, Nuts, Wheat germ, Whole grains. Herbs: Alfalfa, Dandelion, Wheat Grass, Yellow Dock.

Vitamin B6 • 1.5-2 mg • Water-soluble vitamin	Nervous system, mental wellness, healthy skin, mineral balance, prevents fluid retention before menstruation, blood cell formation, pregnancy, antibody produciton, aids synthesis of RNA and DNA.	Skin disease, mental problems, arteriosclerosis, PMS, Carpal Tunnel, anemia, seizures, sore tongue, nervousness, depression, irritability, abdominal pain, weak immune response.	Generally considered nontoxic. High doses (2,000-6,000 mg) can cause nerve disorders.	Bananas, avocados, Brewer's yeast, brown rice, whole wheat, peanuts, walnuts, oats, carrots, sunflower seeds. Herbs:Alfalfa, Catnip, Oatstraw.
Vitamin B7 *Biotin* • 25-35 mcg • Water-soluble vitamin	Aids metabolism of macronutrients for energy, especially important to pregnant and nursing mothers, increases health of hair, skin and nails.	Dry, scaly skin or skin rashes, brittle hair, hair loss, fatigue, loss of appetite, insomnia.	Generally nontoxic. Well tolerated in doses up to 200 mg/day (nearly 7,000 times the AI) even in people with hereditary disorders of biotin metabolism.	Dandelion greens, Mushrooms, Spinach, Whole grains. Herbs: Alfalfa, Dandelion, Kelp, Parsley, Wheat Grass.
Vitamin B9 *Folate [Folic Acid, Folacin, Pteroyglutamic Acid (PGA)]* • 400-1,200 mcg • Water-soluble vitamin	Builds red blood cells growth of cells healing, skin, hair (gray hair). Prevents pregnancy-related anemia. Regulates production, division and maintenances of new cells. Vital for nourishing the brain. Strengthens the immunity and is used for energy production.	Anemia, irritability, weakness, sleep disturbances, pallor, sore and reddened tongue.	Folic acid greater than 1 mg daily might cause abdominal cramps, diarrhea, rash, sleep disorders, irritability, confusion, nausea, stomach upset, behavior changes, skin reactions, seizures, gas, excitability, and other side effects.	Asparagus, Barley, Beer, Bran, Brewer's Yeast, Broccoli, Brown rice, Brussels Sprouts, Dates, Green Leafy Vegetables, Legumes, Lentils, Spinach, Mushrooms, Okra, Oranges, Pinto Beans, Split Peas, Whole Grains.

Vitamin B10 *Para Aminobenzoic Acid (PABA)* • 20-100 mg • A basic part of Folate • Water Soluble Vitamin-like substance	Aids utilization of Pantothenic Acid. An antioxidant. Converted to folate by intestinal bacteria. Aids intestinal flora, flexibility of muscles. Decreases inflammation of joints and skin. Prevents hair loss. Aids in the formation and utilization of protein.	Eczema, infertility, senility, wrinkles, fatigue, loss of pigmentation, arthritis, gastrointestinal problems, anemia, lupus, premature gray hair, hair loss.	Generally considered nontoxic. Toxicity occurs at doses above 1200 mg and are usually a result of over-supplementation. Toxicity causes liver, kidney and blood problems.	Brewer's Yeast, Mushrooms, Spinach, Whole Grains. Herbs: Alfalfa, Dandelion Leaves, Kumbu.
Vitamin B12 *(Cyanocabalamin, Cobalt)* • 25-500 mcg • Water-soluble vitamin	Red blood cell growth and production, enzymes actions, iron absorption, increases memory, restful sleep, fertility, metabolism of macronutrients.	Unsteady gait, chronic fatigue, constipation, depression, digestive disturbances, dizziness, drowsiness, mood swings, pernicious anemia, spinal cord degeneration.	Generally considered nontoxic.	Alfalfa Sprouts, Bananas, Bee Pollen, Brewer's Yeast, Seeds, Soybeans, Wheat Germ. Herbs: Alfalfa, Bladderwrack, Catnip, Comfrey, Dong Quai, Dulse, Hops, Kelp, Spirulina.

Vitamin C • 60-5,000 mg • Water-soluble vitamin	Protects against all diseases and infections, Increases health of glands and organs. Reduces stress, asthma symptoms. Antioxidant, antiviral. Healthy teeth, gums and skin.	Poor wound healing, bleeding gums, tooth decay, easy bruising, fatigue, nosebleeds, joint pain, edema, frequent colds and infections, anemia, scurvy.	Generally considered nontoxic. High doses >5,000 mg daily) can case abdominal bloating and diarrhea.	Avocados, Asparagus, Broccoli, Cantaloupe, Cherries, Collard Greens, Dandelion Greens, Grapefruit, Kale, Kiwi, Lemons, Limes, Mangos, Mustard Greens, Onions, Oranges, Papaya, Peppers, Persimmons, Pineapple, Strawberries, Radishes, Star fruit. Herbs: Alfafa, Bonoset, Catnip, Chickweed, Oregano, Pokeweeds, Dandelion, Hibiscus, Marigold, Watercress.
Vitamin P *Bioflavenoids* • 200-250 mg • Water-soluble antioxidant	Regulate cellular activity, fight free radicals, prevents cancer. Good for heart health and inflammation. Anti-viral and anti-allergy.	Easy bruising, hemorrhaging, inflammation, arthritis, diabetes, asthma, allergies, eczema, hemorrhoids, infections, hypertension	Generally considered nontoxic, even at high doses.	All Fresh Fruits and Vegetables, Apricots, Blackberries, Black Currants, Broccoli, Buckwheat, Cherries, Citrus Fruits, Grapes, Hot Peppers, Kale, Red Onions, Rutabaga, Spinach. Herbs: Chervil, Elderberries, Harthorn Berry, Horsetail, Rosehips, Shepherd's Purse, Watercress.

Minerals				
Boron	Builds strong bones and muscles, increases testosterone levels. Improves thinking skills and muscle coordination. Helps metabolize fats, sugars, calcium, magnesium and phosphorus.	Cancer of the lungs and reproductive organs, impaired brain function, osteoporosis, arthritis, poor wounds healing.	Problems of the stomach, liver, kidney, intestines and brain.	Apples, Carrots, Grapes, Raw Nuts, Pears, Green Leafy Vegetables, Whole Grains.
Calcium • 1,000-1,500 mg • Mineral	Formation and health of bones and teeth, nerve transmission, cellular adhesion, muscle, excitement and contraction, blood coagulation, Regular heartbeat and nerve signals, lowers cholesterol and blood pressure. Maintains cell membrane permeability, healthy skin, calming effect, relieves cramps, relaxes smooth muscle and aids respiratory system.	Soft bones, decay, nervousness, mental problems, muscle spasms, cramps, high blood pressure, brittle nails, eczema, high cholesterol, numbness, arthritis, heart problems, rickets, osteomalacia, osteoporosis.	Upset stomach, abdominal pain, nausea, vomiting, and constipation. Bone pain and muscle weakness. Hypercalcemia can cause the bones to release too much calcium, leaving them deficient.	All Leafy Greens, Almonds, Asparagus, Beans, Broccoli, Brussels, Sprouts, Cabbage, Carob, Collard Greens, Dulse, Figs, Hazelnuts, Kale, Millet, Mustard Greens, Oats, Okra, Prunes, Rutabaga, Sesame Seeds, Soy Beans, Turnip Greens, Walnuts. Herbs: Cayenne, Chamomile, Chives, Parsley, Flaxseeds, Fenugreek Red Clover, Sorrel, Watercress.

Chloride • 98-106 mEq/L • Mineral	Maintains the balance of fluid inside and outside the cells, proper blood volume, blood pressure, pH of body fluids.	Fluid loss, dehydration, weakness or fatigue, difficulty breathing, diarrhea, vomitting	Fatigue, muscle weakness, excessive thirst, dry mucous membranes, high blood pressure	Seaweed, Rye, Tomatoes, Lettuce, Celery, Olives. Found in many foods combined with potassium, such as in Sea Salt.
Choline • 200-600 mg • Mineral	Essential for digestion. Aids in nerve and brain function, and metabolizing fats. Good for memory. Helps form hormones. Minimizes excess liver fat.	Anxiety, restless-ness, fatty liver, muscle damage, cancer, hemorrhag-ic kidney necrosis, hyperhomocyste-inemia	Hypotension, excessive sweating, salivation, fishy body odor, gastrointestinal diarrhea, nausea and vomiting.	Asparagus, Avocado, Beans, Cabbage, Celery, Cucumber, Dandelion, Endive, Kale, Oats, Pineapple, Spirulina, Tomatoes, Turnips, Whole Grains. Herbs: Betony, Burdock, Kelp, Nettle, Spirulina.
Chromium *(taken as chromium picolinate or GTF chromium)* • 200-600 mcg • Essential Trace mineral	Blood sugar control, regulation of carbohydrates in the cells, digestion of protein and glucose metabolism of fats and cholesterol. regulates levels of manganese. Heart function, vital during pregnancy.	Diabetes, low blood sugar, heart disease, hardening of arteries, anxiety fatigue, alteration of metabolism of fats, carbohydrates, proteins, and amino acids.	Generally considered nontoxic; exposure to industrially inhaled chromium has been linked to lung cancer.	Beer, Brewer's Yeast, Broccoli, Brown Rice, Corn, Grape Juice, Mushrooms, Potatoes, Wine, Whole Grains. Herbs: Alfafa, Catnip, Dulse, Kelp, Licorice, Nettle, Spirulina, Yarrow, Wild Yam.

Copper • 1.5-3 mg • Mineral	Maintains healthy joints and nerves. Aids in formation of antioxidants. Aids in digestive enzyme formation. Creates blood cells and collagen, which is needed for connective tissue, bones and skin.	Anemia, fatigue, frequent sickness, weak and brittle bones, memory loss and learning problems, difficulties walking, pale skin, sensitivity to cold, premature gray hair, baldness, skin disease, liver problems.	Headaches, fever, fainting, vomiting, blood in vomit, diarrhea, black stools, abdominal cramps, jaundice.	Beans, Dark Chocolate, Fruits, Leafy Greens, Raw Nuts and Seeds, Shitake Mushrooms, Whole Grains.
Germanium • Trace mineral	Assists in getting oxygen to body's tissues. Increases white blood cell function and boosts immune system. Reduces pain. Helps body excrete toxins.	Cancer, immune system dysfunction, heart disease, osteoporosis.	Nontoxic.	Brocoli, Celery, Garlic, Mushrooms, Radish, Onions, Rhubarb, Tomatoes. Herbs: Aloe Vera, Comfrey, Ginger Root, Ginseng.
Iodine • 150-300 mcg • Mineral	Essential for regulation of mental and physical activity, helps the skin, thyroid and aids fat metabolism. Used in the production of thyroid hormones, which help to regulate metabolism and growth during pregnancy.	Growth and sexual development delays in children, goiter, fatigue, anemia, breast cancer, low blood pressure, loss of sexual activity	Generally considered nontoxic under 1, 000 mcg daily; high doses can cause headaches, metallic taste in mouth, and rash, doses over 20,000 mcg daily have been associated with iodine goiter.	Asparagus, Garlic, Lima Beans, Mushrooms, Seaweed, Sesame Seeds, Spinach, Swiss Chard, Squash, Turnip Greens. Herbs: Black Walnut Hulls, Dulse, Jojoba, Kelp, Sarsaparilla, Sea Moss, Watercress.

Iron • 15-25 mg (men) • 18-30 mg (women) • Mineral	Creation of hemoglobin, helps hemoglobin hold oxygen in the blood. creates red blood cells (with B12 and folic acid), important for physical and brain development, energy production, important for enzymes.	Mental problems, nervous disorders, anemia, tired, fatigue, prior resistance to disease, pale complexion, headache, brittle hair, digestion problems, dizziness, long menstruation, candidiasis, arthritis, herpes.	Generally considered nontoxic if taken under 75 mg daily; high doses can cause abdominal cramps, vomiting, and diarrhea, severe overdoses of iron can be fatal if medical attention is not sought.	Almonds, Apricots, Avocados, Bananas, Beans, Beets, Brown rice, Lentils, Millet, Peaches, Pears, Prunes, Pumpkins, Raisins, Rye, Sesame Seeds, Spinach, Sunflower Seeds, Turnip Greens, walnuts, Winter Squash, whole grains. Herbs: Alfalfa, Burdock Root, Cayene, Chamomile, Chickweed, Dong Quai, Fenugreek, Kelp, Parsley, Sarsaparilla, Shepherd's Purse, Yellow Dock, Watercress.
Lithium • Trace mineral	Vital for nerves and brain.	Mental problems such as depression, nervous disorders, schizophrenia, and bi-polar disorder.	Toxicity can occur with prescription medication. Symptoms include nausea, vomiting, diarrhea, tremor, dysarthria, nystagmus, ataxia, and slurred speech.	Sea Water, Natural Mineral Spring Water. Herbs: Kelp.

Magnesium • 280-350 mg • Mineral	Promotes mineral absorption. Helps bone formation. Aids in digestive enzyme activity. Metabolizes carbohydrates. Dissolves kidney stones. Reduces cholesterol levels. Stabilizes nerves and aids nerve signal transmission. Reduces muscle cramps.	Nervousness, depression, seizures, irritability, confusion, rapid heartbeat, insomnia, asthma, fatigue, poor digestion, lung problems, bone loss, diabetes	Hypotension, nausea, vomiting, facial flushing, urine retention, muscle weakness, irregular heartbeat, extreme	Avocados, Dark Chocolate, Apples, Apricots, Bananas, Nuts and Seeds, Legumes, Figs, Garlic, Green Leafy Vegetables, Whole Grains, Millet, Lemons, Cantaloupe, Sesame Seeds, Black Eyed Peas, Soybeans. Herbs: Alfalfa, Dandelion Root, Lemon Grass, Nettle, Parsley, Peppermint, Sage, Yellow Dock.
Manganese • 2-5 mg • Mineral	Necessary for bone formation, digestion, nerves, brain, blood sugar regulation, reproductive muscles and immunity. Needed for protein and fat metabolism. Used in the formation of synovial fluid found in joints and cartilage.	Digestive problems, asthma, poor libido, confusion, memory loss, convulsions, tremors, tooth grinding, eye problems, hardening of the arteries, heart problems, hypertension.	Permanent neurological damage including tremors, walking difficulties, facial muscle spasms. May experience irritability, aggressiveness and hallucinations.	Apricots, Avocados, Beets, Blueberries, Brussels sprouts, Garlic, Grapefruit, Nuts and Seeds, Oranges, Peas, Pineapples, Spinach, Green Leafy Vegetables, Whole Grains. Herbs: Alfafa, Burdock Root, Chickweed, Dandelion, Parsley, Yarrow, Yellow Dock.

Molybednum • 0.075-0.250 mg • Trace Mineral	Necessary for protein synthesis. Helps normal cell function. Aids teeth and. Bone growth. Stimulates enzymes.	Retarded growth. Mouth and gum disease. Impotence in older men.	Rare; usually only occurs by way of oversupplementa-tion.	Beans, Spinach, Dark Leafy Greens, Whole Grains, Legumes, Peas.
Phosphorus • 700 mg (adults) • Mineral	Strengthens teeth and bones, helps make energy, move muscles, filters waste from kidneys, growth and repair of tissues and cells, produces genetic building blocks DNA and RNA, maintains a regular heartbeat, facilitates nerve conduction	Joint or bone pain, loss of appetite, irritability, anxiety, fatigue, poor bone development in children.	Joint pain, muscle pain, muscle weakness. Itching, red eyes, constipation, nausea, vomiting, diarrhea.	Amaranth, Beans, Brazil Nuts, Cashews, Dried Fruit, Lentils, Sunflower Seeds, Pumpkin Seeds, Pine Nuts, Pistachios, Potatoes, Quinoa. Herbs: Alfalfa, Dulse, Kelp, Marigold, Rosehips, Rosemary, Sorrel, Watercress.
Potassium • 3,500-4,700 mg • Mineral	Bone health, blood pressure regulation, normal water balance, muscles contractions, nerve impulses, digestion, heart rhythm, pH balance	High blood pressure, kidney stones, bone turnover, urinary calcium excretion, salt sensitivity, constipation, extreme fatigue, muscle weakness, cramping, malaise	Heart arrhythmias, chest pains, numbness, tingling, difficulty breathing, nausea	Bananas, Cantaloupe, Cucumbers, Dates, Grapefruit, Honeydew, Mushrooms, Oranges, Peas, Potatoes, Prunes, Raisins, Spinach, Sweet Potatoes. Herbs: Catnip, Dandelion, Dulse, Eyebright, Horsetail, Hops, Nettle, Parsley, Rosemary, Skullcap, Watercress.

Selenium • 40-70 mcg/day • Mineral	Liver and thyroid function. Prevents certain tumors. An antioxidant. Prostate health. Aids against cataracts, high blood pressure, infertility, cancer, arthritis and lung problems.	Infertility in men and women, muscle weakness, weakened immune system, hair loss, liver problems, digestive problems, infections, heart disease, pancreas problems, cancer	Nausea, vomiting, hair loss, nail discoloration and brittleness, irritability, fatigue, foul breath	Brazil nuts, Broccoli, Brown Rice, Garlic, Onions, Mushrooms, Herbs: Alfalfa, Burdock Root, Catnip, Chamomile, Ginseng, Kelp, Spirulina, Nettle, Parsley, Sarsaparilla, Yellow Dock.
Silicon • Mineral	Protects against weak bones. Maintains flexible arteries. Prevents heart disease. Aids formation of connective tissue and collagen. Maintains healthy hair, skin and nails.	Bone problems, stiff joints, infections, weak connective tissue, mental problems, skin impurities, itchy skin, dull split hair.	Generally non-toxic.	Barley, Beets, Brown Rice, Bells Peppers, Dark Leafy Green Vegetables, Oats, Soy Beans, Whole Grains. Herbs: Horsetail

Sulphur (Includes MSM) • Mineral	Nourished hair, skin and nails. Resists bacteria and disinfects the blood. Guards against effects of radiation and pollution. Needed for the synthesis of amino acids Cysteine, Glutathione, Methionine and Taurine.	Skin problems, blemishes, rashes, split ends in hair, weak brittle nails, gastrointestinal problems, slow wound healing.	Low toxicity. May cause gas, bloating, headaches, brain fog and tiredness in those with sulfur sensitivity.	Brussels sprouts, Cabbage, Celery, Kale, Garlic, Onions, Plantain, Soybeans, Turnips, Wheat Germ. Herbs:Eyebright, Horseradish, Horsetail, Irish Moss
Vanadium • Mineral	Aids growth and reproduction. Essential for insulin production. Aids in sugar, lipid and cholesterol metabolism. Builds strong bones and teeth. Lowers cholesterol.	Bone deformities, growth retardation, infertility.	Gastrointestinal symptoms such as vomiting, diarrhea and weight reduction. Liver and kidney problems.	Beer, Black Pepper, Mushrooms, Olives, Radishes, Snap Beans, Whole Grains. Herbs: Dill, Parsley.

Zinc	Cell growth; sexual maturation; night vision; mobilization of vitamin A from liver (converts retinol and then to retinoid acid): in the body, over 200 enzymes require zinc as a catalyst.	Impaired sexual functions, acne, hair loss, high cholesterol. recurrent colds, white spots on toe and/ or fingernails, poo sense of taste and smell, hair growth problems, slow healing, poor resistance to disease, impotence, fatigue, memory problems.	Symptoms include nausea, vomiting, abdominal pain, impaired coordination, fatigue.	Kelp, Nuts, Legumes, Lima beans, Mushrooms, Pecans, Pumpkin and Sunflower Seeds, Soybeans, Wheatgerm.
• 22-50 mg • Mineral				

Amino Acid	Function	Natural Food Sources
Essential Aminos Acids **Vital to human life and cannot be produced in the body, so you need to get them from food sources.**		
Histidine (His)	Allows for erection by relaxing penis sponge tissue. Improves female orgasm. Metabolized into histamine. Protects against radiation. Treats rheumatoid arthritis and allergies.	Navy beans, Squash Seeds, Pumpkin Seeds. Tofu, Whole grains
Isoleucine (Ile)	Treats chronic mental and physical illness.	Brazil nuts, Beans, Black Eyed- Peas, Brown Rice, Raw Peanuts, Tofu, Whole Wheat

Leucine (Leu)	Used to treat mental and physical illness of all kinds.	Almonds, Brazil nuts, Beans, Carrots, Chickpeas, Lentils, Lima Beans, Mushrooms, Raw Peanuts, Pumpkin Seeds, Sesame Seeds, Soybeans (cooked), Strawberries, Tomato (raw), Walnuts, Whole Wheat Bread, Wheatgerm.
Lysine (Lys)	Antiviral. Used to treat herpes simplex infection. Helps make Carnitine. Helps with skin problems. Improves concentration. Treats symptoms of tired blood-fatigue, anemia, dizziness.	Brown Rice, Carrots, Chickpeas, Lentils, Nuts and Seeds, Oatmeal, Orange, Peach, Potato, Soybeans (cooked), Soyaflour, Tomato (raw), Wheatgerm.
Methionine (Met)	An antioxidant. Aids thyroid function. Treats depression, atherosclerosis and fatty liver. Heavy metal detoxification. Needed for the synthesis of Taurine, Cystine and Cysteine.	Almonds, Brazil nuts, Mushrooms, Orange, Peach, Pumpkin Seeds, Raw Peanuts, Soybeans (cooked)
Phenylalanine (Phe)	Aids in weight loss and depression. Helps with pain. Stimulates Tyrosine, a precursor of dopamine.	Almonds, Carrots, Chickpeas, Lentils, Potato, Pumpkin Seeds, Sesame, Soybeans (cooked),
Threonine (Thr)	Essential for the nervous system. Used to treat mental problems.	Beans, Brazil nuts, Brown Rice, Peaches, Oatmeal, Potato, Pumpkin Seeds, Sesame Seeds, Soybeans (cooked), Wheatgerm
Tryptophan (Trp)	Enhances brain function, stimulates serotonin, induces sleep and emotional calmness. An antidepressant. Reduces carbohydrate cravings and aides weight loss.	Avocado, Bananas, Broccoli, Brown Rice, Brussels Sprouts, Cantaloupe, Corn, Dates, Grapefruit, Pineapple, Plantains, Soybeans, Tomatoes.
Valine (Val)	Enhances energy, increases endurance. Aids in muscle tissue recovery and repair. Lovers elevated blood sugar levels. Increases growth hormone production.	Mushrooms, Oatmeal, Peanuts, , Podded Peas, Raw Nuts and Seeds, Soy, Whole Grains.

Conditionally Essential Amino Acids		
Can be synthesized in the body, but in certain circumstances you need to get them from food.		
Arginine (Arg)	Aids thymus activity and fat metabolism. Increases wound healing. Chelates manganese. Helps infertility caused by poor movement of sperm.	Lentils, Nuts and Seeds, Peanuts, Pumpkin Seeds, Sesame Seeds, Spirulina, Sunflower Seeds, Watermelon, Whole Grains.
Carnitine (Car) • **Synthesized from lysine and methionine.**	Metabolizes fats and decreases triglycerides. Improves circulation and sperm mobility. Prevents heart attacks and heart death. Helpful against muscular dystrophy.	Asparagus, Avocado, Beans, Legumes, Nuts and Seeds, Whole Grains.
Cysteine (Cys)	Removes heavy metal deposits. Helps stabilize insulin. Helps build enzymes. Protects against effects of alcohol and smoking. Maintenance of hair, skin, nails and detoxing of free radicals.	Legumes, Lentils, Oatmeal, Sunflower Seeds.
Glutamine (Gln)	An energy source for intestinal and immune cells. Aids in proper growth of intestinal cells.	Beans, Beets, Brussels sprouts, Carrots, Celery, Kale, Miso, Papaya, Parsley, Spinach, Whole Wheat.
Glycine (Gly)	Needed for the growth and maintenance for tissue, and for making hormones and enzymes.	Brazil Nuts, Legumes, Nuts, Seeds, Spirulina.
Ornithine (Orn) • **Synthesized from arginine through the urea cycle.**	Stimulates growth hormone. Aids weight loss. Absorbed through the intestinal tract and incorporated into liver, kidney and skeletal muscle. Aides body in the removal of waste.	Beans, Legumes, Lentils, Peanuts, Pumpkin Seeds, Soybeans, Spirulina, Quinoa, Whole Grains.
Proline (Pro)	Used to make collagen, which is necessary for the connective tissue and support of the skeletal system. Plays an important role in wound healing and immune responses. Promotes digestive health, contributes to a healthy metabolism and fights inflammation.	Asparagus, Bell Peppers, Broccoli, Cabbage, Citrus Fruits, Kamut, Mushrooms, Strawberries, Soy.

Tyrosine (Tyr)	A precursor of thyroid hormones and the neurotransmitters dopa, dopamine, norepinephrine and epinephrine. Important for health of the brain and neurological system. Used to treat depression and Parkinson's disease.	Almonds, Avocados, Bananas, Lima Beans, Pumpkin Seeds, Sesame Seeds.
Non-essential Amino Acids **Produced in the body, even if we do not get it from food.**		
Alanine (Ala)	Lowers cholesterol. Essential in metabolizing Tryptophan and Vitamin B6. A source of energy for the muscles and nervous system. Strengthens the immune system.	Brown Rice, Nuts, Seaweed, Soybeans, Whole Grains.
Asparagine (Asn)	Helps transfer amino acids in the liver. Aides in making glycoproteins. Required for brain development and function. Detoxes body of ammonia. Increases endurance in athletes.	Asparagus, Legumes, Nuts, Seeds, Potatoes, Whole Grains.
Aspartic Acid (Asp)	Helps transfer amino acids in the liver. Aides in making glycoproteins, which have numerous physiological functions, including immunity. Detoxes body of ammonia. Increases endurance in athletes.	Asparagus, Bamboo Shoots, Kidney Beans, Lentils ,Red Peppers, Seaweed, Spirulina, Spinach, Soy, Watercress.
Citrulline • **Derived from arginine.**	Aids in detoxification from drug use. Helps arteries to relax. Aides in good stamina by increasing blood flow to muscle mass. Combats fatigue. Plays a vital role in the urea cycle.	Present in many foods, especially Bitter Melon, Cucumber, Gourds, Pumpkin and Watermelon.
Gama Aminobutyric Acid (GABA) • **Formed from Glumatic Acid with Vitamin B6.**	Stimulates prolactin. Used in the treatment of nerve damage and mental illnesses Induces calmness in manic mental conditions such as anxiety, panic disorders and Attention Deficit Hyperactivity Disorder. Stabilizes nervous system. . Treats seizures and and movement disorders such as Parkinson's disease.	Almonds, Beans, Berries, Brocoli, Citrus Fruits, Coca, Fava Beans, Lentils, Nuts, Potatoes, Sunflower Seeds, Walnuts, Tomatoes.

Glutamic Acid (Glu) • **Derived from Glutamine.**	Nourishes the muscles. Treats nerve damage. Gives energy to the brain. One of the main amino acids found in cerebrospinal fluid. Increases memory. Helps to produce GABA, which calms the brain. An anti-depressant. Decreases addiction and alcoholism. Improves circulation. Relieves peptic ulcers.	Almonds, Nuts, Peanuts, Pumpkin Seeds, Seaweed, Sesame Seeds, Soy, Squash Seeds, Sunflower Seeds, Watermelon Seeds, Whole Wheat.
Selenocysteine (Sec) • **Produced from cysteine.**	A building block of selenoproteins (selenium containing proteins), which act as enzymes. Important for fundamental cellular processes, including maintaining selenium homeostasis. Maintains the overall metabolic rate. Can be converted into glucose.	Brazil nuts, Corn, Rice, Oats, Walnuts, Whole Wheat.
Serine	Used in moisturizing creams and cosmetics to hydrate the skin. Plays and important role in protein synthesis and intracellular metabolism. Inhibits brain inflammation.	Almonds, Asparagus, Bamboo Shoots, Chickpeas, Kidney Beans, Edamame, Lentils, Horseradish (raw), Nuts, Seaweed, Soybeans, Spinach, Spirulina, Watercress, Zucchini Squash.

Low vibration foods

Poor quality foods, GMOs, artificial foods and food-like products.
Little to no nutritional value.
Produce emotional, mental and physical imbalance in the body.
Create an acidic, dis-eased internal environment.
Eliminate from diet for optimal health.

Devitalized Carbohydrates

- Commercially grown fruit and vegetables (generally sprayed with toxic pesticides)

- Canned fruits and vegetables

- Frozen entrees

- Seedless fruit

- Deep-fried vegetables

- Artificial bread and baked goods

- Commercial cereals

- White flour products

- Instant noodles

- Instant rice

- Instant oatmeal and breakfast cereals

- White rice

- White sugar

- Enriched white pasta

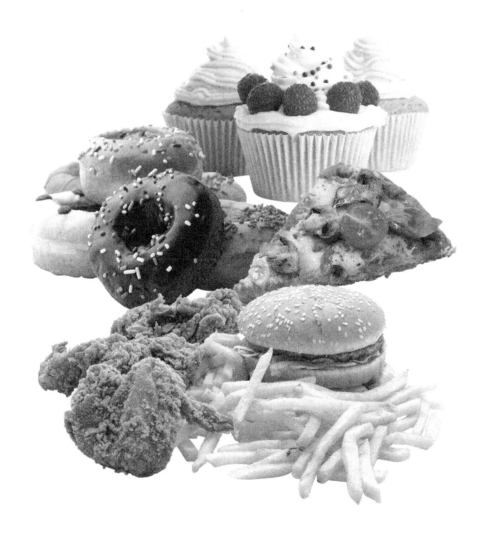

Poor Quality Proteins

- Milk: Cow or goats milk including 1% milk, 2% milk, skim milk, half & half, dairy creamers

- Dairy products (ex: butter, cheese, yogurt, ice cream)

- Canned milk products: condensed milk, evaporated milk

- Boxed milk (UHT milk)

- Artificial dairy products: powdered creamer, margarine, artificial cheese products

- Animal flesh: beef, pork, goat, lamb, chicken, eggs, fish, shellfish, etc.

- Canned meat (ex: chicken, corned beef, tuna, crab)

- Farm-raised fish

- Imitation meat or fish such as spam, imitation crab meat and fish sticks

- Deli/lunch meats

- Cured meats: bacon, corned beef, hot dogs, salami, sausages, prosciutto, pork, etc.

- Fast food meat products

- Fried or barbecued meat

- Microwaveable meat products and T.V. dinners

- Canned beans/legumes

- Soy food products: genetically engineered soy foods, soy supplements, and soy junk foods like soy cheese, soy ice cream, soybean oil, soy burgers, and soy meat-substitutes

Fats

- Commercial vegetable oils such as corn oil and canola oil (made from GMO corn and canola)
- Lard
- Partially hydrogenated oils such as in:
- Margarine
- Vegetable shortening
- Packaged snacks
- Commercially baked foods
- Ready-to-use dough
- Coffee creamers (dairy and non-dairy)
- Cooking spray
- Fried foods
- Transfats

Liquids

- Alcoholic beverages
- Animal's Milk (cow, goat)
- Artificial fruit juices
- Energy drinks
- Instant Coffee
- Soda
- Sugary Drinks
- Tap water

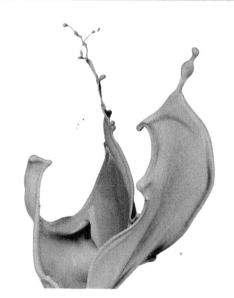

Commercial Spices and Sweeteners:

- Artificial sweeteners
- Artificial flavor bouillons
- High fructose corn syrup
- Ketchup
- Commercial mayonnaise
- MSG and artificial flavor enhancers
- Pancake syrup
- Table salt
- White sugar

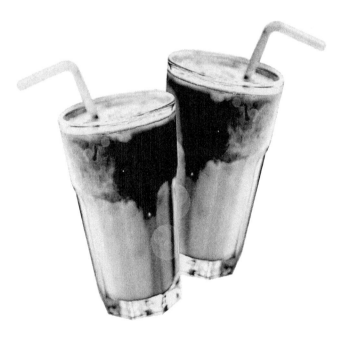

GMOs

Genetically engineered

Low vibration imitation food

What are GMOs?

The term GMO stands for Genetically Modified Organisms. These are food products containing living organisms whose genetic material has been artificially manipulated in a laboratory through gene-splicing or genetic engineering. These food-like substances have been altered at the gene (DNA) level. Essentially GMO's are food-like lab creations. Because these substances are not natural, they are not recognized by the body and can have detrimental effects on your health.

Which foods contain GMOs?

Over 80% of all packaged foods in the supermarkets contain GMO's, and the FDA does not require labeling of these foods. The most commonly modified foods in the U.S. are corn, soybean, cotton, canola (rapeseed), sugar beets (used to make refined sugar), alfalfa and papaya. Packaged foods with these ingredients very likely contain GMOs. Meat, fish and dairy also have genetically engineered ingredients. Chickens and cattle are raised in unsanitary conditions, injected with hormones to make them bigger and pumped with antibiotics when they get sick from their filthy conditions. Tumors found in the meat from diseased animals are cut out, and the meat is packaged and sold. Milk from these cows contain pus and growth hormones. The pasteurization of milk purportedly makes it "safe" for consumption while also yielding a nutritionally dead product. GMO salmon is labeled as "farm-raised."

How do I avoid GMOs?

Because the FDA does not require companies to inform consumers that their products contain GMOs, you must read the product labels and beware of common GMO ingredients. With few exceptions, all major fast-food products contain GMO ingredients. When shopping, buy whole foods that are not packaged or processed. Packaged products should be labeled USDA Certified Organic or Non-GMO Project Verified (see images below). Shop at farmer's markets. Avoid seafood or fish labeled "farmed-raised." Instead, purchase wild-caught fish. Reduce your consumption of meat. It is best to purchase meat from a local butcher or farmer's market. Know where your food is coming from. Always buy organic dairy. Chicken and eggs should be labeled cage-free, hormone-free, antibiotic-free and/or organic. Beef should be avoided unless organic and grass-fed. Animal milk, if consumed, should be purchased organic only.

Look for these labels on your packaged foods:

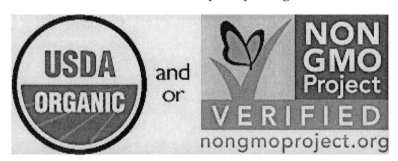

Know Your Labels

Read PLU number on your produce, which indicates how the produce was grown. Conventionally grown fruits and vegetables, grown using the full array of modern agricultural chemicals and pesticides, has a 4-digit PLU number. Organically grown fruits and vegetables have a 5-digit PLU number starting with 9, which indicates organically grown produce. GMOs, genetically modified/ genetically engineered, fruits and vegetables also have a 5-digit PLU number starting with 8, indicating genetically engineered produce.

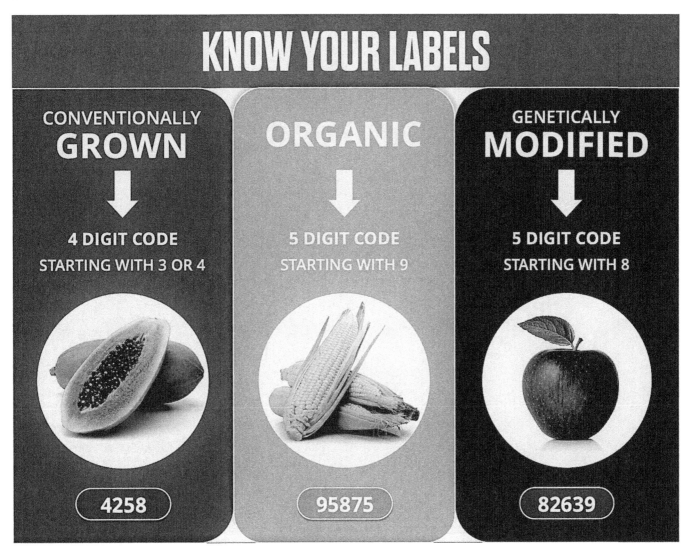

KNOW YOUR LABELS

CONVENTIONALLY GROWN	ORGANIC	GENETICALLY MODIFIED
⬇	⬇	⬇
4 DIGIT CODE STARTING WITH 3 OR 4	5 DIGIT CODE STARTING WITH 9	5 DIGIT CODE STARTING WITH 8
4258	95875	82639

COMMON GMO'S TO AVOID

Packaged products with the ingredients listed below are likely genetically engineered unless labeled "USDA Organic" or "Non-GMO Project Verified" and should be avoided:

Aspartame (Aminosweet, Nutrasweet, Equal, Sweet N' Low)	Glycerin	Oleic Acid
Baking Powder	Glycerol	Phenylalanine
Canola Oil (Rapeseed Oil)	Glycerol Monooleate	Phytic Acid
Caramel Color	Glycine	Protein Isolate
Cellulose	Hemicellulose	Shoyu
Citric Acid	High Fructose Corn Syrup (HFCS)	Sorbitol
Cobalamin (synthetic Vitamin B12)	Hydrogenated Starch	Soy Flour
Colorose	Hydrolyzed Vegetable Protein	Soy Isolates
Condensed Milk	Inositol	Soy Lecithin
Confectioners Sugar	Inverse Syrup	Soy Milk
Corn Flour	Inversol	Soy Oil
Corn Masa	Invert Sugar	Soy Protein
Corn Meal	Isoflavones	Soy Protein Isolate
Corn Oil	Lactic Acid	Soy Sauce
Corn Sugar	Lecithin	Splenda
Corn Syrup	Leucine	Starch
Cornstarch	Lysine	Stearic Acid
Cottonseed Oil	Malitol	Sugar (unless specified as cane, coconut or date sugar)
Cyclodextrin	Malt	Tamari
Cystein	Malt Syrup	Tempeh
Dextrin	Malt Extract	Teriyaki Marinades
Dextrose	Maltodextrin	Textured Vegetable Protein
Diacetyl	Maltose	Threonine
Diglyceride	Mannitol	Tocopherols labeled with a dl– prefix (synthetic Vitamin E)
Erythritol	Methylcellulose	Tofu
Equal	Milk Powder	Trehalose
Food Starch	Milo Starch	Triglyceride
Fructose (Any Form)	Modified Food Starch	Vegetable Fat
	Modified Starch	Vegetable Oil
		Whey

HIGH VIBRATION NUTRITION ALTERNATIVES

Low Vibration Food & Food-like Products	High Vibration Nutrition
Artificial fruit juices	Organic, fresh fruit juice
Animal flesh (chicken, beef, fish, etc)	Avocado, mushrooms, legumes (sprouts, beans, nuts, seeds), jackfruit, seitan
Butter/ margarine	Vegan butter spread, coconut oil, cold pressed olive oil
Candy	Fresh or dried fruit
Cheese	Vegan cashew cheese, nutritional yeast
Chocolate	Cacao, carob, dark chocolate
Commercial vegetable oil (canola, corn oil)	Cold-pressed olive oil, coconut oil, grapeseed oil
Cow or goats milk	Plant-based milk (almond, coconut milk, etc)
Eggs (scrambled)	Sauteed ackee
Eggs (in baked goods)	Vegan egg replacer or apple sauce
Heavy cream	1:1 ratio of water to pureed tofu or 2/3 cup almond milk (or other plant-based milk) + 1/3 cup oil
Ice cream	Almond or coconut ice cream. Fruit sorbet. Frozen blended fruit.
Pancake syrup	Organic pure maple syrup
Soda	Fruit infused sparkling water
Table Salt	Dulse, kelp, Himalayan pink salt, liquid aminos, sea salt, vegetable bullion
Tap Water	Natural spiring water, distilled water
White bread	100% whole grain or sprouted bread
White flour	Whole wheat flour. Gluten free: almond flour, coconut flour, cornmeal
White rice	Brown rice, wild rice
White sugar	Agave, raw honey, black strap molasses, dates, pure maple syrup
Yogurt	Coconut or almond yogurt

ALKALINE-ACID BALANCE

The pH of human blood should be slightly alkaline (7.35 to 7.45) to maintain the balance of the body systems (homeostasis). Above or below this range creates an environment for disease formation. A ph of 6.4 to 6.9 is neutral. Below 6.4 pH is acidic and above 7 pH is alkaline. An acidic state causes a lack of oxygen at the cellular level, which leads to dis-ease. The Standard American Diet (SAD) is high in acidic foods such as meat, dairy and processed foods and low in detoxifying, alkaline foods. The fastest way to balance pH is with food. An optimal diet consists of all-natural, organic foods eaten in a balance of 80% alkaline to 20% acid foods. To create a healthy internal environment, avoid altogether low-quality animal flesh, dairy, artificial foods, white flour and white sugar products.

Food Combining

No matter our dietary lifestyle, the combination of foods must be in Ma'at (balance, harmony and right order). Food combining is one of the most important, yet rarely discussed, components in eating for proper nutrition.

The body goes through four stages in breaking down food: ingestion, digestion, absorption/assimilation and elimination. All stages are key in maintaining digestive wellness and balance in bodily functioning. Ingestion is the intake of food into the alimentary canal. Digestion is the breaking down of food. Once food is broken down, it can be absorbed and used for the functions of the body (assimilation). Finally, the removal of waste and toxins occurs via elimination (urination and defecation).

Digestion of the three main macronutrients (carbohydrates/starches, proteins, and fats) begins in the mouth through chewing and salivary enzymes. Carbohydrates are broken down by the enzyme amylase, which begins in the mouth and continues in the stomach and small intestines. Lipase begins the breakdown of fats in the mouth, which continues in the stomach. Fats are further broken down by lipase and bile in the small intestines. Protein digestion begins in the stomach, facilitated by the enzyme pepsin. Trypsin and chymotrypsin continue protein digestion in the small intestines. Food passes from the small intestines to the large intestines, where water is absorbed from the indigestible food matter, and the waste material is released from the body.

Digestive issues arise from poor quality foods and improper food combining. The body's digestive enzymes work to break down food particles to be used for nutrients in cellular function. Based on their biochemical composition, different foods require different lengths of time and different enzymes for proper digestion.

Water and other liquids, for example, are easily assimilated into the bloodstream and typically digest within 15 minutes. Denser foods require more time to process. Fruit is best eaten alone 30 to 60 minutes before meals, as the enzymes in fruit do not combine well with other foods. Vegetables and other starches take 1-3 hours to digest. Leafy Greens combine well with all foods (except fruit). Starches do not combine well with heavy proteins because they require different biochemical environments for breakdown. When the two are eaten together, the proteins are digested first, leaving the starch to ferment in the stomach during the extended digestion time.

Animal flesh (chicken, beef, seafood, etc.) takes the longest time to digest, typically 4 to 8 hours. The extended digestion time allows the meat to putrefy within the digestive tract, causing indigestion, bloating, foul-smelling bowels and overextended bellies. For those who choose to eat meat, it is best eaten alone or with greens for proper digestion. Fats (coconut oil, olive oil) combine well with vegetables and grains. Avoid large amounts of fats with protein, as in the mayonnaise in a tuna casserole, for example.

ALKALINE			ACIDIC		
Highly Alkaline pH 9.5 to 10.0:	Moderately Alkaline pH 8.5 to 9.0:	Mildly Alkaline pH 7.5 to 8.0:	Slightly Acidic to Neutral pH 6.5 to 7.0	Moderately Acidic pH 6.0 to 5.5:	Extremely Acidic pH 5.0 to 3.0:
Alfalfa	Avocado	Almonds	Amaranth	Bread, refined	Alcohol
Barley Grass	Beet Greens	Apple	Barley Black beans	Butter	Artificial fruit juice
Bee Pollen	Beets	Apricot	Blueberries	Cheese	Artificial sweeteners
Broccoli	Chard Greens	Banana	Cashews	Corn and rice	Aspirin
Cantaloupe	Carrot	Chestnuts	Corn	breads	Beef
Celery	Celery	Chili Pepper	Cranberries	Eggs	Canned/Glazed Fruits
Chlorella	Collard Greens	Cinnamon	Currants	Mustard	Chicken
Cucumber	Dates, dried	Coconut, fresh	Dried beans	Pasta, whole grain	Cigarrettes
Daikon	Eggplant	Currants	Dried fruit	Rice, brown	Coffee
Dandelions	Fermented	Curry	Honey	Wheat Germ	Corn syrup
Dulse	Figs, dried	Fresh Fruit Juice	Maple Syrup	Whole wheat foods	Drugs, prescription & OTC
Garlic	Ginger	Grapes, seeded	Oils		Drugs, recreational
Green Juices	Grapefruit	Herbs (all)	Olives		Fast foods
Honeydew	Molasses,	Lettuce	Peanut Butter		Fish
Kale	blackstrap	Millet	Peanuts		Flour, white
Lecithin	Vegetables	Mineral Water	Pecans		Fried foods
granules	Green Beans	Mushrooms	Plums		Goat
Lemon	Mustard Greens	Mustard	Prunes		Instant foods
Lime	Okra	Nectarine	Rye		Lamb
Melon	Onions	Orange	Spelt		Microwaved meals
Parsley	Parsnips	Peach	Walnuts		Pasta, refined
Probiotic	Peppers	Pear			Rice, white
Cultures	Radishes	Pineapple			Soda
(dairy free)		Peas			Sugar
Pumpkin		Pumpkin			
Seeds		Quinoa			
Sea Salt		Raisins			
Sea		Raspberries			
Vegetables		Rutabaga			
Spinach		Sweet Potatoes			
		Stevia			
		Strawberries			
		Tamari			
		Tangerine			
		Tomato			
		Tropical Fruits			
		Watercress			

DIVINE FOOD COMBINING

Food	Digestion Time	Divine Combining
Water	0-10 minutes	Drink alone 10-15 minutes before or after meals.
Liquids	15-30 minutes	Drink alone 15-30 minutes before or after meals.
Fruits acid (lemons, limes, oranges, grapefruit) sub acid (apples, berries, cherries, mangos, peaches) sweet and dried fruit (bananas, dates, grapes, raisins) melon (cantaloupe, honeydew, watermelon)	30-60 minutes	Eat fruit alone 30-60 minutes before meals. Sub-acid fruit combine well with acid and sweet fruit. Acid fruit and sweet fruit do not mix well with each other. Melons are best eaten alone. Citrus and dairy do not mix.
Vegetables Leafy greens (spinach, arugula) Starchy vegetables (yam, plantains, cassava) Fermented Foods (pickles, kimchi, sauerkraut) Grains (amaranth, barley, quinoa)	1-2 hours	Leafy Greens combine well with most foods. Complex carbohydrates and starchy vegetables eaten with animal protein slows digestion, making them a poor combination. Fermented foods combine well with most vegetables, complex carbohydrates and concentrated proteins. Avoid eating with foods high in sugar and fat.
Vegetable Protein Legumes (beans, nuts and seeds)	2-3 hours	Combine well with greens and vegetables of all kinds.
Animal Protein Animal milk (cow, goat, etc.) Dairy products Fish, chicken, beef, pork	4+ hours	Meat is best eaten with greens or alone. Concentrated proteins combine poorly with heavy starches (ex: cheeseburger on a bun).
Fats Oils & butters Nuts and seeds	4+ hours	Avoid combining large amounts of fat with concentrated proteins (ex: mayonnaise in tuna casserole).

ELIMINATION

Elimination is an essential part of the digestive process, which is often ignored when considering overall health and wellness. Waste is formed with the digestion of every meal. If you are not eliminating, you are retaining. Studies show that most American adults retain between 5 and 25 lbs. of fecal matter in the intestines and colon. The average American consumes 3-5 meals per day but has only 3 bowel movements per week. This is severe constipation and it is not natural or healthy! As this toxic waste builds up, the body begins to experience fatigue, weight gain, digestive issues (IBS, gastric reflux), chronic skin conditions (acne, eczema), brain fog, mental changes (mood swings, anxiety, depression).... and that's just the beginning!

A typical Western diet is high in sugar, meat and starch, while low in fiber. This is a recipe for chronic constipation. It takes quite a few hours for animal flesh to makes its way through our digestive systems. This extended digestive period allows the meat to putrefy as it sits in the digestive tract. The ammonia by-product of this putrefaction can also be toxic. Poor quality starches such as white bread and pasta also impair healthy elimination. Because starch is a binder, foods high in starch content slow down bowel movements causing constipation. Natural foods high in water content and fiber are most beneficial to proper digestion and healthy elimination patterns.

Create Healthy Elimination Patterns	Causes of Impaired Elimination
• Diet high in chlorophyll-rich, high fiber foods such as green leafy vegetables, tubers, fruit and whole grains. Helpful foods include berries of all kinds, grapes, kiwi, papaya, pears, plums, prunes, apricots, kale, spinach, swiss chard, cabbage, green beans, squash, zucchini, barley, and oats.	• The Standard American Diet (SAD), which is high in constipating foods such as sugar, salt, starch, processed foods and meat.
• Daily exercise stimulates the natural contractions of muscles in the intestines, assisting the body in expelling food waste.	• Diet low in chlorophyll-rich and high fiber foods such as green leafy vegetables, fruit and whole grains.
• Proper hydration. Your daily water intake should equal half your body weight in ounces. For example, a 140 lb. person should be consuming at least 70 oz. (or 8.75 cups) of water per day.	• Lack of physical exercise hinders peristalsis (the forward movement of food through the digestive tract).
• Fruits and vegetables with high water content (watermelon, cucumber, celery, etc.) hydrate the body and flush waste from the digestive system.	• Dehydration. The large intestine will reabsorb water from your food waste if the body is dehydrated, contributing to hard and infrequent bowel movements.
• Gelatinous foods such as okra, aloe vera, chia seeds, psyllium husks, flax seeds, slippery elm, seaweed lubricate the GI tract and have fibers that help to sweep the intestines clean.	• Over consumption of alcoholic and caffeinated beverages. These substances dehydrate the body, further contributing to constipation. For each cup of alcoholic or caffeinated beverage, two cups of water must be consumed to compensate.
• 2 tsp. Black seed oil or castor oil taken orally twice a day can ease the passage of excrement from the colon.	• Many over the counter, prescription and recreational drugs can lead to constipation. These include anti-depressives, antacids containing aluminum, calcium and iron, antihistamines, narcotics and other pain killers, some high blood pressure and Parkinson's disease medications.
• Herbal teas such as senna, anise and fennel tea have laxative properties that ease constipation.	

Cultural Nutrition:

Your healing is in your culture.

Food is cultural and your stomach has a culture too. When choosing foods for optimal nutrition, it is essential to take into account your genetic background. It takes over 2,000 years for the stomach culture of a species to change. This means that the foods typically eaten by your ancestors will also be the healthiest for you, even if you are living in a different part of the world than your ancestors' indigenous land.

The climate and topography of the land affect the cultural diet of the people on the land. Historically, African people were sedentary. Most were farmers with land who planted their own food. They raised their own goats, cattle, chickens and sheep. Therefore the foods they consumed were natural foods from the land and from the animals they raised. Euro-Asiatic groups were nomadic. They ate what they could find. The diet is a reflection of the culture.

The natural foods for those of African heritage include fresh plant foods such as fruits and vegetables of all kinds, herbs and various ground provisions like yams and sweet potatoes. Healthy traditional diets of African ancestry include greens like spinach, collards, mustard and turnip greens, which help to cleanse the blood, liver and kidneys. Disease amongst African descendants in the global diaspora such as diabetes, heart disease, asthma, cancer and obesity were quite rare when they were eating from the land. However, as Africans have adopted a Western diet, their health has severely declined.

Case Study:

In a study conducted in 2015 at the University of Pittsburgh, 20 African Americans and 20 South Africans switched diets for two weeks. During this time, the South Africans consumed a Standard American Diet (SAD)—high in meat, cheese and starch and low in vegetation—while African Americans took on a traditional African diet—high in fiber and low in fat, with plenty of vegetables, beans, and cornmeal, with little meat.

After the exchange, researchers performed colonoscopies on both groups and found that those in the African diet group increased the production of butyrate, a fatty acid proven to protect against colon cancer. Members of the American diet group, on the other hand, developed changes in their gut that scientists say precede the development of cancerous cells. What was even more astounding to Dr. Stephen J. O'Keefe was that the diet changes produced microbiota that was cancerous within just two weeks in the Africans.

---

[1]MacMillan Publishers Limited (2015). "Fat, fibre and cancer risk in African Americans and rural Africans." https://www.nature.com/articles/ncomms7342 . Nature Communications, Accessed 6 September 2016.

Examine the major cultural and climatic regions around the world. Discover how topography and climate affect people, vegetation, and consequently, the diet and nutrition of the people in each respective region.

African Origins of Human Life and Migration

In "African Time (Universe to 1896) EXPANDED EDITION", Dr. Ife Kilaminanjaro *et al.* outlines:

> Initially, all modern humans originated on the north-south axis of eastern Africa between 150,000 and 200,000 years ago, and moved into the rest of the globe between 85,000 and 30,000 years ago. The peopling of North, South, and Central America was merely the initial northeastern-most expression of this process. Born in Africa, on the equator, in an extremely hot and temperate climate, all human life was initially Black before it migrated to other parts of the world and adapted to other climates.

> Essentially, then, the origins of the earliest humans in the Western Hemisphere trace back to Asia in the same way the Asians and Europeans ultimately trace their origins back to Africa. Humans began in one place, Africa, and became different in skin, hair and eye color as they migrated out of Africa to different parts of the world.

> Asians then migrated from Asia into what became called Beringia, Alaska, and then into what is now called North America, proceeding west to California, south to New Mexico, east to New York and Pennsylvania, and southeast into Florida, Georgia and Texas. These Asian populations adapted phenotypically to the environments they migrated into. (Fagan 1989, p.32-51 cited Ife Kilamanjaro *et al.* 2020, p. 455)

African Diaspora

The African diaspora is a term that refers to the present-day Black Africans living on and off the African continent. This consists of the worldwide collection of communities descended from indigenous Black Africans who have settled in different regions throughout the Americas and the Caribbean, either by way of human migration or the Transatlantic slave trade. Africans were world travelers, settling in the Americas, the Caribbean, Europe and Asia long before the slave trading of African people.

Most African peoples lived agrarian lifestyles, eating from the cultivation of the land, fish and livestock. Many foods that are home to the African continent are ingrained in the cultural diet of African people, wherever they may be in the world. Across Africa, couscous, sorghum, millet, and rice were enjoyed as the bases of meals or as porridges and sides. Watermelon and okra are both native to Africa, and many believe that cucumbers are too. Beans were eaten in abundance everywhere, especially black-eyed peas, which were often pounded into a powder for tasty bean pastes or seared as fritters. Africa is home to leafy greens, root vegetables, mashed tubers and beans, and many different plant crops across its lands.

North Africa

[Includes Algeria, Kemet (Egypt), Libya, Morocco, Sudan, Tunisia, Western Sahara]

- North Africa's climate is primarily arid desert land with mountainous regions and fertile plains irrigated by rivers and seacoasts. The Atlas Mountains, which extend across much of Algeria, Morocco and Tunisia, encompass a vast complex of plains and plateaus. The mountainous regions also receive the highest amounts of rainfall.

- Daily high temperatures of 122 °F (50 °C) are not uncommon in the Sahara, while winters are cool with daily temperatures of about 55 °F (13 °C).

- Water is the chief factor in determining where and how people of North Africa live. In Kemet, 95 percent of the people live within a short distance of the Nile River, whose waters irrigate fields of cereal grains, vegetables, cotton, and other crops.

- Vegetables made up a major part of the ancient Kemetic diet. Many foods were eaten raw or sun-cooked as opposed to stove cooking. Wheat was not a major part of the diet. Spelt, especially as loaves of bread, was eaten instead. Natural wine and beer were consumed on rare occasions and in small quantities and were primarily made from barley. Some types of birds and fish, especially those considered sacred, were eaten raw, either sun-dried or salted. They also ate quails, ducks and other small birds raw after picking them in brine. Other types of birds and fish were prepared by roasting or boiling. Papyrus reeds, lotus flowers and other lilies were also prepared as food.

- In the other North African countries, about 90 percent of the people live within 200 miles of the coast, generally in valleys with streams and rivers. The arid conditions of the desert make farming nearly impossible, except in oases, where the main crops raised are date palms, fruit, and cereal grains. Other major crops include citrus fruits, olives, and grapes. The waterways make these areas suitable for agriculture, especially with the aid of irrigation.

- Farther south, where hills and grasslands border the desert, is home to the indigenous Nilotic tribes of the Nile Valley region. These are primarily pastoralist tribes who raise herds of sheep, goats, cattle, and camels; and whose diets consist mostly of dairy products, including milk and blood, with some meat, and varying percentages of vegetables. They presently inhabit South Sudan, Sudan, Ethiopia, Uganda, Kenya, the Democratic Republic of Congo and Tanzania.

- Present-day North African cuisine has been usurped by the culture and religion of Arab invaders from West Asia. Arabic North Africa is known today for its Tagine stews comprised of mixed vegetables served over couscous. Foods are often flavored with aromatic herbs such as hot chilies, parsley, basil, tomato paste, cumin, caraway, turmeric and nutmeg, ginger, saffron, and paprika. Chickpeas and white beans are common ingredients, as are stews of lamb, fish, and beef. Dried fruits like figs, apricots, prunes and raisins are often included in meat dishes.

Central and West Africa

[Includes Angola, Central African Republic, Cameroon, Chad, Congo, Ghana, Guinea, Ivory Coast, Liberia, Nigeria and Rwanda]

- Central Africa's terrain ranges from the tropical rainforests in Chad to the mountainous regions of The Congo. Characterized by uninhabited jungle rainforests, bush and game reserves.

- Most of West Africa has only one rainy season, which lasts between one and six months, with uniformly high sunshine and high temperatures. West African terrain contains a broad range of habitats, from rain forest to desert. Temperatures in the lowlands are generally above 65 °F (18 °C). Maximum temperatures in the Sahel can reach 104 °F (40 °C).

- Principal food crops include cassava, peanuts, sorghum, millet, maize, sesame and plantains. Main cash crops include cotton, coffee, and tobacco.

- West Africa is home to some of the world's most delicious tropical fruits, including mango, avocado, banana, apple, pineapple, pawpaw (papaya), guava, coconut, tangerine, lemon, grenadilla, puts, breadfruit, malombo, soursop, sweetsop, sapodilla, star apple, baobab fruit and black tumbler.

- Known for hearty vegetable soups and stews, full of spices and aromas, poured over boiled and mashed tubers or grains.

- Many dishes are enriched with a base of onions, tomatoes and chili peppers.

- The most popular cooking oil is palm nut oil.

- Common cooking ingredients include ginger, maize, rice, millet, peanut, tamarind leaves, Baobab fruit, sorghum, fonio, okra, black-eyed peas, sesame, kola nuts, egusi seeds, guinea fowl, and melegueta pepper.

East Africa

[Includes Ethiopia, Eritrea, Kenya, Madagascar, Somalia, Tanzania, Uganda and Zimbabwe]

- East Africa's geography is dominated by the Great Rift Valley, extending through the middle of the region from the north to south. Associated with the rift valleys are vast savannas such as the Serengeti Plain, large lakes, high mountains and the highlands of Ethiopia. Eastern Africa consists largely of plateaus and has most of the highest elevations in the continent, particularly in Ethiopia and Kenya.

- Temperatures in East Africa are moderate with highs of around 77 °F (25 °C) and lows of around 59 °F (15 °C), except along the hot and generally humid coastal belt.

- Whole grains and vegetables are the main features of traditional meals, especially cabbage, kale and maize (cornmeal).

- Traditional meals are based on flat-breads like *injera* (made out of teff, sorghum or whole wheat) and beans like lentils, fava beans, and chickpeas blended with spices.

- Due to Arabic influence, many meals in the Horn of Africa (where Ethiopia and Somalia are found) are prepared in halal style, meaning that they include no pork, no alcohol, and meat only from animals who have died on their own.

Southern Africa

[Includes South Africa, Mozambique, Namibia, Swaziland, Lesotho and Botswana]

- Geographic features of Southern Africa include grasslands, savannas, sub-tropical woodland, forest, desert, shrubland, mountainous regions, rain forests, beaches and coastal wetlands. Mozambique is noted for its coastal lowlands with uplands in its center and high plateaus in the northwest. The climate is tropical with two seasons— summer and winter. Lesotho boasts a scenic land of tall mountains and narrow valleys, with a negligible percentage of its land covered with water. Desert covers approximately 70% of Botswana's surface, which is mostly flat with a few hills.

- Summer (October- April) is the rainy season in South Africa, ranging in temperature between 59 °F and 97 °F. Winter (June to August) temperatures fall between 28 °F (-2 °C) and 79 °F (26 °C), depending on the altitude and location.

- Southern Africa is bordered by the South Atlantic Ocean, the Indian and the Antarctic Ocean.

- Indigenous grain crops include amaranth, pearl millet, sorghum, cowpea, bambara groundnut, mungbean, and marama bean. Vegetable crops include roots and leafy vegetables such as cleome, cowpea, amaranth, blackjack, Jew's mallow, cassava, amadumbe, and marama bean. Indigenous fruit crops include marula, sour plum, monkey orange and sour fig.

- Cookery practices by the indigenous people, such as the Sotho and Nguni- speaking people, were comprised of a wide range of foods, including fruits, nuts, bulbs, leaves and other products gathered from wild plants and hunting wild game.

- Primary food staples include cooked grains, especially sorghum, fermented milk (somewhat like yogurt) and roasted or stewed meat. At some point, maize replaced sorghum as the primary grain.

- Modern-day cuisine has been influenced by European colonizers such as the Dutch, German, French, Italian, Greek and British and their Indo-Asian slaves. Cooking styles from neighboring colonial cultures such as Portuguese Mozambique have also influenced South African cuisine.

African American

[Refers to the Foundational Black Americans who built the United States of America from scratch.]

- North America's geography can be classified into forests, coniferous forest, mediterranean, grassland, tundra, alpine, rainforest and desert. Climate and temperatures vary according to the region. For example, Northern U.S.A. experiences four different seasons with warm to hot summers and cold, wet, snowy winters. Meanwhile, the Gulf and South Atlantic states have a humid subtropical climate with mostly mild winters and hot, humid summers.

- Foundational Black Americans, a term coined by American activist Tariq Nasheed, refers to Black American Natives who settled here long before European contact, and to the descendants of the Black people who survived the atrocity of the American slave trade. Africans brought over by Spanish colonizer Lucas Vázquez de Ayllón in 1526, were the first documented foreign settlers in the New World of North America. They arrived along with 600 Spaniards in the area now known as the South Carolina/Georgia coast. The enslaved Black people revolted from their Spanish captives, forcing the remaining Spanish terrorists back towards the Caribbean. Once liberated, they amalgamated into the local Native American society, forming what would later become African American culture.

- Traditional African American foods came straight from the garden, such as cabbage, okra, tomatoes, peppers, and greens were abundant, including dandelion, mustard, collards, and turnip greens.

- Pickling vegetables was a popular way to preserve food. This includes pickled beets, radish, cabbage, carrots, and cucumbers were enjoyed—and the list goes on.

- Louisiana's Creole cooking has its roots in French, Spanish and Haitian cuisines, with a common base called "The Holy Trinity": celery, onions and red bell peppers all equally chopped—which is at the heart of Louisiana's popular Gumbo soup.

- Traditional Low Country cooking, from South Carolina and Georgia's coast, features oysters, crabs, shrimp, sweet potatoes, Hoppin' John, and rice.

Afro-Caribbean

[Includes Antigua, Barbuda, Bahamas, Barbados, Belize, Cuba, Dominican Republic, Grenada, Haiti, Jamaica, St. Kitts and Nevis, St. Vincent, the Grenadines, Suriname, Trinidad and Tobago]

- There are more than 700 Caribbean islands, which are located in North America, southeast of the Gulf of Mexico, east of Central America and north of South America.

- The climate of the Caribbean is tropical, varying from the tropical savanna to the tropical rainforest. Temperatures are generally warm to hot year-round.

- There is a dry season, which runs from about February to June, and a wet season between July and January.

- Approximately 23 million people of African descent live in the Caribbean along with Taino Natives, French, Spanish and Indo-Asian peoples.

- The Caribbean Islands bring tropical accents and various seafood elements like cod and conch.

- Rice and peas, featuring pigeon peas or red beans, are typically served with any of the various locally found meats such as beef, poultry, mutton, pork or fish.

- Common spices and flavorings include annatto, coconut milk, garlic, onions, scotch bonnet peppers, celery, scallions, ginger, cilantro, chives, marjoram, rosemary, tarragon and thyme. These spices are used for a variety of dishes like curries, stews and roasted meats.

- Tropical fruits include ackee, avocado, banana, breadfruit, coconut, custard apple (cherimoya), guava, jackfruit, june plum, naseberry (sapodilla), papaya, passion fruit, mango, pineapple, plantain, star apple, star fruit (carambola), stinkingtoe, soursop, sugar cane, sweetsop, tamarind and watermelon.

- Callaloo, cassava, chocho (chayote), cocoa bean, dasheen (taro), green banana, Irish moss (sea moss), okra, yam, sorel, and sweet potato are all commonly grown vegetation in the Caribbean islands.

- In the southern parts of the Caribbean, roti is a popular flat-bread, primarily made from whole wheat flour, that can be filled with curried vegetables and shrimp, or bean dishes, as a warm, soft roll-up.

Afro-South American

- There are an estimated 100 million people of African descent living in South America, with a large majority in Brazil.

- The African presence in the Americas dates back as early as approximately 800 BCE. Many were also brought to the Americas during the 15th-century transatlantic slave trade.

- South America's climate is dominated by relatively warm regions, yet the continent can generally be grouped into 4 zones: tropical, cold, dry and temperate.

- Geographical features include rain forests with jungles of dense wet forests, desert regions, deciduous forests, grasslands, savannas and mediterranean regions.

- Native food crops include maize (corn), potatoes, quinoa, *canahua*, several species of beans, tubers such as *ullucu* and *oca*, squashes, pumpkins, cashews, brazil nuts, and cacao.

- Bananas, mangoes, oranges, lemons and grapefruits are grown widely throughout South America.

- Soups and stews are very popular, as are rice and beans, and tubers like yucca and cassava.

- Okra, peanuts, squashes, and plantains appear on many plates, often accompanied by fruits and fruit juices like mangoes and guava.

- A few favorite ingredients are red snapper, avocado, cilantro, and tapioca.

- Native American roots are seen in their corn/maize use and their tamales that combine peas, carrots, potatoes, rice, and various spices as filings.

- Moqueca Baiana is a popular traditional dish in Brazil. It is a seafood stew with prominent African roots made using palm oil, coconut milk, shrimp and crab, onions, garlic, peppers, tomatoes, and cilantro.

Asia

Vegetables such as bamboo shoots, bean sprouts, bitter melon, boy choy, broccoli, cabbage, daikon, eggplant, kumquats, leeks, lemongrass, mushrooms, peppers, pumpkins, scallions, seaweed, snow peas, spinach, sweet potatoes and yams are common ingredients in Asian cuisine. Rice is the staple grain in Asia, which produces over 90% of the world's rice. Principal cash crops include tea, spices, palm oil, coconuts and sugarcane. Apricots, bananas, cherries, coconut, dates, dragon fruit, kiwi, lychee, mandarins, mangoes, milk fruit, oranges, papaya, rambutan and tangerines are all widely grown and eaten in a number of Asian countries.

Central Asia

[Includes Tajikistan, Uzbekistan, Kazakhstan, Turkmenistan and Kyrgyzstan]

- Central Asia is known for its distinctive arid (desert) and semi-arid climate, having little or no rain, and too dry or barren to support vegetation.

- Due to arid conditions that produce little to no natural vegetation, Central Asia is primarily a nomadic culture. Cooking techniques and major ingredients are influenced by their nomadic way of life. Nomads eat whatever is near, traditionally, this meant horse, goat or sheep meat and dairy.

- Signature dish is *palov*, made with rice, pieces of meat, carrots and onions.

- Meals are traditionally served with naan, a flatbread.

- Local agriculture includes a large amount of grain farming, so bread and noodles are major staples. Other common crops include chia, wheat, barley, maize, rice, dairy products (mainly yogurt), various nuts and native vegetables, fresh and dried fruits (grapes).

East Asia

[China, Hong Kong, Japan, Mongolia, North Korea, South Korea, Taiwan, Tibet and Macau]

- Eastern China has a humid subtropical climate--cool winters and hot summers with plenty of rain. Temperatures are lower towards the North with warm summers and cold winters.

- South Korea and Japan are mostly surrounded by water. Therefore, summers are a bit cooler and winters are a bit warmer than other places at the same latitude.

- The northern interior of China, on the other hand, is very dry, with arid and semiarid climate regions. Temperatures there can range from very hot to very cold. The Plateau of Tibet, located to the south of China, has a highland climate with cool to cold temperatures.

- Many diverse seafood and woodland delicacies are used, including a myriad of fish, shellfish and turtles, along with edible mushrooms and bamboo shoots.

- Many dishes include live seafood, fats, oils and sauces. Rice and wheat noodles are also quite popular.

- Traditional regional cuisines rely on basic methods of food preservation such as drying, salting, pickling and fermentation.

- Northern styles feature oils and strong flavors derived from ingredients such as vinegar and garlic, while Southern styles tend to favor fresh ingredients that are lightly prepared.

- Pork, chicken and seafood are favored proteins, supplemented by a wide variety of soy products. Vegetables add nutrients, flavor and color to dishes, with a wide array of cabbages, greens, onions, sprouts and mushrooms put to good use.

South Asia

[Includes Afghanistan, Bangladesh, India, the Maldives, Nepal, Pakistan and Sri Lanka]

- The climate of South Asia can be divided into three climates: tropical, dry and temperate.

- Nepal, Bangladesh and Bhutan Northeast region where temperatures range between warm and tropical to subtropical (temperate) climates. The Western region, where Afghanistan and Pakistan are located, is known for it's dry, desert climate.

- South Asian food is heavily influenced by Indian cuisine. Foods are flavored with a wide variety of strong herbs and spices including chili peppers, black peppers, cardamom, cinnamon, clove, coconut, coriander, ginger, fenugreek, and mustard seeds, along with flavored butter and ghee.

- Curried vegetable dishes of all varieties are made using turmeric and cumin.

- Common meats include lamb, goat, fish and chicken. Beef is less common than in Western cuisines because cattle are sacred in the Hindu religion, which dominates this area of the world.

- Prohibitions against beef extend to the meat of cows and yaks. Pork is considered a taboo food item by all Muslims and is avoided by some Hindus.

Southeast Asia

[Includes Cambodia, Indonesia, Laos, Malaysia, Philippines, Singapore, Thailand, Vietnam]

- A region of peninsulas and islands, which includes beaches, bays, inlets and gulfs. The climate of Southeast Asia is hot and humid and can be described as tropical, with the exception of The Myanmar Himalayas and North Vietnam, which both have subtropical climates.

- There is a strong emphasis on lightly prepared dishes with a robust aromatic component. Spices and flavors include citrus and herbs such as mint, cilantro (coriander leaves) and basil. Ingredients also include the use of flavors such as galangal, tamarind and lemongrass. Soy sauce is more commonly used than the fish sauce of East Asian cuisine.

- Cooking methods include a balance of stir-frying, boiling and steaming.

- Local foods include tropical fruits, rice, noodles, drinks, dessert and various soups.

- Cuisine is characterized by Portuguese, Dutch, British, Chinese, Malay, Indian and Peranakan influences.

West Asia

[Referred to in present-day to as the Middle East, this region includes Armenia, Azerbaijan, Bahrain, Cyprus, Georgia, Iraq, Iran, Jordan, Kuwait, Lebanon, Qatar, Saudi Arabia, Syria, and Yemen]

- Primarily arid and semi-arid climate, and can be subject to drought. Deserts regions yield infertile lands and scarce agriculture. Some areas of grasslands, rangelands, mountains, forests and fertile valleys. Major rivers such as the Tigris and Euphrates provide irrigation for agriculture.

- Main crops include wheat, barley, chickpeas, maize, fava bean, sunflower, sesame seeds and lentils. Primary livestock includes sheep, goats, cows and camel.

- Tahini, a sesame paste made with hulled seeds, is a staple ingredient in many Middle Eastern dishes. It is featured in many popular West Asian appetizers such as baba ghanoush and hummus, along with pungent dipping sauces served with falafel, keftes or kofta and vegetables.

- Hummus is made from chickpeas, which are staples of the diet. Some commonly used ingredients include olives and olive oil, lamb, pitas, honey, sesame seeds, dates, sumac, chickpeas, mint and parsley.

- Red meat is eaten frequently, as in some popular dishes such as kibbeh and shawarma (sliced lamb).

- Arab cuisine of the Persian Gulf today is the result of a combination of diverse cuisines incorporating Lebanese, Indian, Chinese, and Persian cooking styles, and many items not originally indigenous to the Persian Gulf region, which were most probably imported on the dhows and the caravans.

- Primary crops are dates, bananas, citrus fruits, pomegranates, mangoes, cucumbers and tomatoes.

North Asia

[Siberia, Ural or the Russian Far East. Also known as Northwest Asia or Eurasia]

- The climate of Siberia typically has short summers and long, brutally cold winters. Temperatures average about -39 °F but are as low as -69 °F in certain areas.

- Russia's climatic and geographic factors limit agricultural activity to about 10 percent of the total land area. Of that amount, about 60 percent is used for crops, the remainder for pasture and meadow.

- Grains are Russia's most important crops, occupying over 50% of cropland. Primary crops include wheat, barley, corn, legumes, and potatoes. Flax, sunflowers and soybeans are used in the making of vegetable cooking oil. Main fruits and vegetables include sugar beets, carrots, cabbage, tomatoes and apples.

- The cultural diet of North Asia consists of mainly Russian, Yakut (or Sakha) and Yamal cuisine. Buryats also have their own cuisine, although it is very similar to that of the related Mongolians.

- Meat is more prominent and served in larger portions than in other cultures. Cattle are the most common form of livestock, as well as sheep, goats, and pigs. Chicken is kept only in small numbers, and frozen chicken is one of Russia's largest import items.

- Large emphasis on grape wine in the use of cooking as well as sauces as spices and seasonings. Many dairy products are used, especially cheese, which is fermented in many different flavors.

- The most common source of starch is whole wheat bread, as well as pasta, dumplings, patties and potatoes.

Europe

Europe, located in the westernmost part of Eurasia, lies entirely in the Northern Hemisphere and mostly in the Eastern hemisphere. It is generally considered to be separated from Asia by the mountainous Caucus and Ural regions as well as the waterways of the Ural River, the Caspian and Black Seas and the Turkish Straits. Asia borders Eastern Europe, while the Atlantic ocean is to the west, the Arctic Ocean borders the North and the Mediterranean Sea borders Southern Europe. The all-encompassing varied ethnic groups classified as Eurasians have, at times, inhabited the steppes of Central Asia, Mongolia, and what is now Russia. Eurasians are a large group of nomadic peoples from the Eurasian Steppe, who often appear in history as invaders of Europe, Western Asia, East Asia, South Asia and North Africa. Arable land in Europe covers less than one-third of the total surface area. Therefore the European diet generally consists of large servings of meat, poultry or fish accompanied by small side dishes of vegetables and starch. Typical meals are high in protein, mainly from meat and dairy, and low in whole grains, fruits and vegetables.

Northern Europe

[Includes Denmark, Estonia, Finland, Greenland, Iceland, Norway, Sweden, Latvia, Lithuania, and the United Kingdom (which includes England, Great Britain, Wales, Scotland, Ireland)]

- Characterized by humid, cold, snowy winters and mild, cool, humid summers. Northernmost regions such as Iceland, Norway and Sweden have subarctic climates with bitter cold winters and frequent snowstorms. Summers tend to be short with cool, mild temperatures.

- Temperatures in the regions of the United Kingdom have a milder, temperate oceanic climate with cool, wet winters and cool to warm, wet summers. Climate is generally is cool, cloudy and rainy and high temperatures are infrequent.

- Large producers of cereals, roots, edible oils, fibers, fruit, livestock and livestock products.

- Northern European cuisine is well known for its high consumption of meat such as sausage, bacon and ham.

- Onions, cabbage, apples, wheat, barley, chestnuts, wine, and olives are common ingredients in staple dishes.

- Fish, clams, mussels, shrimp and other seafood dishes are customary.

- There is a variety of pastries or dumplings filled with ingredients such as minced meat, potato, cabbage and cheese.

Central and Eastern Europe

[Includes Belarus, Hungary, Moldova, Poland, Romania, Russia, Slovakia, Ukraine]

- Agriculture is mainly divided between crop production and raising livestock. Livestock includes dairy cows, beef cattle, pigs and poultry.

- Main crops include barley, corn, potatoes, sugar beets, wheat and assorted fruits and vegetables.

- Tomatoes, leeks, carrots, corn, cucumbers, endives, lettuce, white cabbage, bell peppers, oat, rye, wheat are mainstays of Eastern European vegetable production.

- Fruit staples include apples, blackberries, blueberries, grapes, gooseberries, kiwis, raspberries, strawberries, and pears.

- Staple dishes include various soups such as *borscht* (a spicy beetroot soup), *paska* (easter bread), dumplings such as *bryndzove halusky* (potato dumplings with sheep cheese and bacon) and *varenyky* (dumpling filled with cheese, mashed potatoes or sauerkraut), and potato pancakes like *draniki* and *lokse*.

Western Europe

[Includes Belgium, France, Germany, Luxembourg, The Netherlands, Switzerland, United Kingdom]

- *Coq au vin* is a very popular dish made with braised chicken cooked in wine, lardons, mushrooms, and garlic.

- Dishes often include meat, cheese and butter with seasonal vegetables. Common ingredients include potatoes, leeks, shrimp, asparagus, endives and beer, cauliflower, Brussels sprouts, lettuce, cucumber, and peppers.

- Fishery of the North Sea river delta gives yield to cod, herring, sole, mackerel, eel, tuna, salmon, trout, oysters, mussels, shrimp and sardines.

- Farming of domesticated animals includes horse, mutton, chicken, cattle, pigs and sheep.

Southern Europe

[Also referred to as the Mediterranean, includes Albania, Bosnia, Bulgaria, Crete, Greece, Spain, Serbia, southern France, Monaco, Portugal, Romania, Italy]

- Three core food elements- olive, wheat, and grapes- yield this region's most popular dishes. Olive oil, bread, pasta and wine are staples of Mediterranean cuisine.

- High quantities of vegetables like tomatoes, kale, broccoli, spinach, carrots, cucumbers and onions are eaten daily.

- Fresh fruit includes apples, bananas, figs, dates, grapes, and melons.

- Legumes, beans, nuts, seeds such as almonds, walnuts, sunflower, seeds and cashews are common ingredients in staple dishes.

- Main starches include whole grains such as wheat, oats, barley, buckwheat, corn, and brown rice.

- Avocado and olives provide healthy sources of fat eaten as is or as olive oil and avocado oil.

- Dairy is frequently consumed, especially in various types of cheese and yogurt.

- Red meats and sweets are limited.

- A drink of one glass of wine per day is common, although water is the main beverage. Carbonated or sweetened drinks are not typically consumed.

- Roast lamb or mutton and meat stews with vegetables and tomato are mainstays in Mediterranean cuisine.

- Influences include the cultural cuisine of Maghreb (of North Africa), Egypt, Levant, Ottoman Empire (Turkey), Greece, Italy and Southern France.

South Pacific (Oceania)

[Oceania is a region centered on islands in the tropical Pacific Ocean, which includes Australia, Cook Islands, Fiji Islands, Hawaii, Tahiti, Indonesia, Melanesia, New Zealand, Polynesia, Samoa, Tonga]

Researchers trace the origins of Pacific Islanders to the first humans to migrate out of Africa approximately 100,000 to 60,000 years ago. During their migration towards East Asia, they made first contact with other hominid species living on the Eurasian landmass before eventually settling and forming their own civilizations in the various islands of Oceania. Polynesians formed a distinct ethnic group with the same basic language and common physical and cultural characteristics. Melanesians and Micronesians include people of many different origins. Unlike the Polynesians, they differ from one another in appearance, physical characteristics, language and customs. The region of Micronesia lies between the Philippines and Hawaii and encompasses more than 2,000 islands. The major islands of Polynesia and Micronesia were settled by about 1300. The islanders had little contact with the outside world until the 1500s, when Europeans began to explore the Pacific.

- The climate of the South Pacific is tropical year-round, with similar weather patterns across all the islands. Temperatures are generally between 72° F (22° C) and 82° F (28° C) and there are only two seasons in the South Pacific. It is warmer and humid from November to April, which is also hurricane season. Temperatures are cooler from May to October.

- A wide variety of tropical foods are grown in this region, including bananas and plantains, betel nut, breadfruit, cassava, coconut, kava, noni, pandanus, sugarcane, sweet potato, taro and yam. The cuisine of each individual island reflects the culture of that particular island.

- Australian indigenous foods are commonly known as 'bush tucker.' Bush tucker comprises a wide variety of herbs, spices, mushrooms, fruits, flowers, vegetables, animals, birds, reptiles, and insects that are native to Australia.

- The cuisine of the indigenous people of these regions has been changed over time due to their influence from European invaders.

- Wild Australian fruits make excellent jams, sauces and desserts. Nuts are used in pies, bread and sweets. New flavors from the bush are making their way into ice-creams, beverages and spices.

- Native Hawaiians fished, raised taro for *poi*, planted coconuts, sugarcane, sweet potatoes and yams, and cooked meat and fish in earth ovens. Modern Hawaiian cuisine has since evolved from their first contact with New England invaders (so-called missionaries) circa 1820.

- Because Pacific Islander diets are based on whole foods found in nature and prepared without excess cooking, the recommended daily amounts of many vitamins and minerals can be met in only one meal. It is only in recent times, with the transition from their traditional diets to imported Western foods, which are highly processed, denatured, low in fiber, and high in fat and refined sugars, that some islanders are beginning to experience nutrition-related diseases such as obesity, type 2 diabetes, and heart disease.

Arctic North America

[The arctic and sub-arctic North American regions including Alaska, Canada and Greenland]

The first human populations of the northernmost regions of North America migrated there in successive waves from Asia across the Bering Sea between 45,000 to 100,000 years ago. Genetically, they are closely related to several northeast Asian ethnic groups from Russia, Siberia and Mongolia.

The topography and climate in the Western Hemisphere include freezing arctic tundra, prairies, miles of mountain ranges, dense rain forests, steppes, swamps, great plains, woodlands, desert shrublands, complex river systems, and freshwater lakes and streams. There are long, cold winters lasting 8-11 months of the year; cool summers and snow is possible year-round. The cold climate makes for short growing seasons, poor soil conditions and difficult agriculture, but a handful of crops that do well. Arctic diets are unique because animal products are staples and plants are seasonal supplements. Diets are traditionally composed of fish and various marine mammals (seals, whales, polar bears), small game, birds, bears, reindeer and plants. Seabird, goose and duck eggs. Typical traditional meals include fresh, boiled, fried or grilled meats, organs and soft bones.

- Common Alaskan grown crops include beets, broccoli, cabbage, carrots, cauliflower, chard, dill, lava bean, garlic, kale, lettuce, parsley, peas, potato, pumpkin, radishes, rhubarb, spinach, snap peas, turnip and zucchini. There are also a slew of berries such as cranberries, salmonberries, raspberries, blackberries, and blueberries.

- Traditional Alaskan cuisine is centered around its cold-water marine life such as crabs, cod, oysters, halibut, whales, seals and especially salmon. Other dishes may include wild game such as moose, reindeer and bears.

- Major field crops grown in Canada include wheat, canola, barley, corn and soybeans. Other crops include rye, oats, white beans and mixed grains. Several specialty crops, which are limited to a very small area of land, are also grown in certain regions.

- In Greenland, plants such as broccoli, radishes, spinach, leeks, lettuce, turnips, chervil, potatoes, parsley, a variety of beans, peas, strawberries and few herbs are grown.

- A variety of beans are grown in Arctic regions of North America, such as lima beans, pole beans, black turtle, pinto, navy, and cranberry beans.

North America and Central America

[The United States of America and the Southernmost regions of North America including Mexico, Honduras, Panama, Costa Rica, Belize, Guatemala, El Salvador, Nicaragua]

Due to the arctic conditions and poor food options in the arctic regions of North America, there was a gradual migration southward throughout the Americas over several generations in different nomadic, hunter-gatherer tribes. Over time, the exploration of uninhabited regions of North and Central America gave way to small groups of Asians, laying the basis for permanent settlements. Through advances in agricultural production, there was a natural increase in nutrition and births and a decrease in mortality. "Between 7,000 BCE and 4,000 BCE, Asians and Africans in America developed agriculture and settled town life based on the cultivation of beans, maize, chili peppers, squash and cotton. They had also begun to domesticate turkeys and ducks." (Ife Kilamanjaro, _et al._ 2020 p. 460)

There are over 1,000 Native American tribes in the United States of America alone. Among the well-known Cherokee, Apache, Navajo, and Iroquois tribes, there are far too many to name in this work. Notable indigenous Central American civilizations include the Aztec, Maya, and the Olmec.

The overall climate of the United States, with the exception of Alaska and Hawaii, is temperate. Summers are generally mild to warm, while winters have cool to cold temperatures. There are 4 distinct seasons with moderate rainfall throughout the year. Temperatures vary depending on the region, with cooler temperatures in the Northernmost regions, warm temperatures in the south, and humid climates in areas closer to the sea. There are eight different climate types in North America, each varying in plant and animal life. Climate types include deciduous forest, coniferous forest, mediterranean, grassland, alpine, desert, and tundra.

- The triad staple crops of Native North and Central American cuisine are corn, squash and beans.

- Other indigenous crops grown include acorns, amaranth, beans, cactus, cashew, cassava, chia, chili and bell peppers, corn (maize), Jerusalem artichoke, papaya, peanut, pecan, peppers, potato, pumpkin, wild rice, dulse seaweed, maple syrup, nuts and seeds, quinoa, strawberry, squash, sweet potato, tomato, tomatillo, sunflower, wild rice, vanilla, and various grains and vegetables.

- Fruits include avocado, black raspberry, blueberry, cacao, chocolate, chokeberries, cranberry, elderberries, guava, papaya, persimmon, pineapple and strawberries.

- Central America's agriculture is known for its vanilla, sugar and spices, allspice, corn, cacao, chocolate, tomatoes, squash, sweet potato, chili and bell peppers.

- Whether they were farmer tribes or not, most Native American tribes had very meat-heavy diets. However, most of their nutrition was derived from nuts and plants. Favorite meats included bison, buffalo, caribou, deer, rabbit, ducks, geese, turkeys and other birds, fish and other marine life such as salmon, clams, shellfish, seals and whales.

South America

[Includes Argentina, Brazil, Bolivia, Chile, Columbia, Ecuador, French Guiana, Paraguay, Peru, Guyana, Suriname, Uruguay, and Venezuela]

Until recently, it was believed that the first human populations of South America, often referred to in Spanish as *pueblos aborigines* (aboriginal people) or *nativos* (natives), settled in the region approximately 14,000 years ago. However, archaeologists today have found sites in South America from Argentina to Chile, ranging between 20,000 to 40,000 years old.

Descendants of indigenous populations of North America who migrated south would become the indigenous populations of South America. The notable Inca empire, emerging in the 13th century, was the largest American civilization prior to Spanish colonization. The South American natives were hunter-gatherers, and indeed many still are, especially in the Amazonian area. Others, especially the Andean cultures, were skilled farmers who utilized advanced agriculture, irrigation and domestication of livestock, such as llamas and alpacas. South America's climate can be divided into seven types: Desert, grassland, deciduous forest, rainforest, savanna, Mediterranean and Alpine. There are four distinct seasons, although temperatures are generally warm to high, especially during the summer months in the desert, grassland, rainforest, Mediterranean and savanna. The grasslands and deciduous forests have cold, wet winters. Alpine regions are known for cold and snowy winters and cool summers.

- South American crops include cassava, lima beans, variety of beans, potatoes, sweet potatoes, tomatoes, guava.

- South Americans typically eat three meals and two snacks daily. Milk is not usually consumed as a beverage but used in coffee, fruit-based drinks and milk-based desserts.

- Coffee is a major beverage throughout the continent, with one-third of the world's coffee produced in Brazil alone. Coffee is consumed most heavily in Argentina, Columbia, Ecuador, and Brazil. Herbal tea, such as the commonly used Yerba mate, is more popular in Chile and Uruguay. Herbal teas are used as remedies throughout the continent.

- Present-day cuisine varies from country to county and tends to blend cultural backgrounds, available foods, cooking styles, and foods of European colonizers. Some regions have a maize-based diet, while others have a rice-based diet. Southern countries Argentina, Chile, Bolivia, Uruguay and Paraguay are major beef producers. Grilled meats such as sides of beef, hogs, lamb, pig, goat, chicken and guinea pig are slow-cooked for hours under layers of hot stones, leaves and herbs, often accompanied by tamales, potatoes and corn.

- Quinoa, or goosefoot plant, is a staple grain in the native South American diet. Its production declined for centuries after the Spanish conquest in the 1500s; however, it is still widely cultivated for its nutritious seeds in Peru, Chile and Bolivia.

- Brazilian foods are a combination of Portuguese, African and native influences. Salted codfish, spicy meat stews and corn or rice pudding desserts came to Brazil through Portuguese invaders. Africans contributed okra, palm oil and peppercorns. Coffee, rum and beer are common beverages. Brazil's national dish, *fejoda completa*, consists of black beans cooked with smoked meats and sausages serviced with rice, sliced oranges, boiled greens and hot sauce topped with toasted cassava meal.

- Columbian and Venezuelan indigenous cuisine has been heavily influenced by their Spanish colonizers. Many foods are served with olive oil, cheese, parsley, cilantro, garlic, onions and chili peppers. Traditional food crops include corn, rice, sorghum, cotton, tobacco, coffee, cocoa, and tubers such as yucca (cassava), potatoes, sweet potatoes and yautia. Legumes include a variety of black, yellow and white beans, including *quinchoncho* (pigeon peas). Vegetables include tomatoes, lettuce, cabbage, carrots, cauliflower, eggplant, cucumber, sisal, beets and peas. A variety of tropical fruits include bananas, plantains, oranges, coconuts and mangoes.

- Guyanese cuisine is a hybrid of African, East Indian, Portuguese, and Chinese influences. Staple foods such as rice and roti are generally served at lunch and dinner. Popular dishes include pepper pot stew, garlic pork, cassava bread, cook-up, and chow mein.

Antarctica

Antarctica is an isolated island, which does not and has never had an indigenous human population. There are no land bridges to Antarctica. This continent was once part of a greater landmass called Gondwana, which included present-day Australasia, Africa, South Asia and South America. Gondwona began to break apart about 180 million years ago. Antarctica split away from Gondwana and settled along the South Pole long before human inhabitants. As its name suggests, Antarctica's climate is arctic with mean annual temperatures of approximately -70° F (-57° C). It is known for being the highest, driest and windiest continent on earth. There are no permanent residents or citizens of Antarctica. Although many people live there for relatively short periods each year, most of them are researchers and scientists. Their stays generally last between 3-6 months, while some last as long as 15 months.

- Because Antarctica is cold and barren, fruits and vegetables are deficient in supply. Fresh produce is shipped via sea or aircraft.

- The majority of foods here are either frozen, dried or canned.

- Commonly eaten foods include *Pemmican*, a combination of ground and dried meat mixed with a large portion of animal fat; *Bannock*, a lightweight bread; *hoosh,* a broth of *Pemmican,* biscuits and melted ice, which is consumed more for sustenance than flavor.

Choose Your Dietary Lifestyle

The four phases of plant-based eating are outlined below to help you in your transition to a high vibration lifestyle that is best for you. Begin at any phase you choose. As you begin to experience the benefits of healthier nutrition, you may choose to move toward a completely plant-based diet. Some people begin a flexitarian or vegetarian diet and advance to a vegan lifestyle over time. Others choose a flexitarian lifestyle with intermittent/seasonal live food detoxing. Choose the nutritional lifestyle that is best for you, eat the most electric, live-giving foods available to assist you in your wellness goals. It is most important and beneficial to consume a natural, plant-based, whole-foods diet free of artificial, genetically-engineered, denatured, food-like products.

Phase I: Flexitarian

This is the beginner stage in plant-based eating. The flexitarian lives a semi-vegetarian lifestyle consisting of a generous intake of live fruits and vegetables, live juices, steamed vegetables, beans, legumes and occasionally organic chicken and fresh water or wild-caught fish. You may choose to go completely meatless for 2-5 days a week. Use the vegetarian menu. You may add chicken or fish where appropriate. Avoid dairy.

Meal Guidelines:

- 50% live foods and 50% cooked foods.

- Live foods include a variety of live fruit and vegetables, soaked nuts and seeds. Liquids include natural spring water, fresh fruit juice, fresh vegetable juice, soup, herbal tea, plant-based milk.

- Cooked foods include a wide variety of vegetables, including legumes and whole grains.

- Plant-based carbohydrates include green leafy vegetables, beans of all kinds, ground provisions, fruits, and whole grains.

- Vegetable sources of protein include various legumes, nuts, seeds, and sea vegetables.

- Vegetable sources of fats include fatty fruits such as avocado and coconut, unrefined nut and seed oils, nut butter, and various nuts and seeds.

- Animal sources of protein and fat include wild caught fish (avoid farm-raised fish), organic cage-free chicken and eggs, organic grass-fed beef, organic butter, ghee and kefir. Consume less than 10% of your protein or fat intake from animal sources.

Phase II: Vegetarian

As a vegetarian, you will be consuming live and steamed vegetables and fruit in generous amounts, omitting all dairy and flesh foods (beef, chicken, fish, etc.). Some vegetarians substitute meat with fermented soy (miso, tempeh, tofu, soy milk, edamame, textured vegetable protein). Others choose to forego the taste of meat altogether with vegetable proteins like beans, sprouts, nuts and seeds. Avocado and mushrooms are also vegetarian favorites for creating fulfilling, hearty meals. As a vegetarian, you will enjoy a much larger portion of live-foods, rather than cooked foods.

Meal Guidelines:

- 50-70% live foods and 30-50% cooked foods

- Live foods include a variety of live fruit and vegetables, soaked nuts and seeds. Liquids include natural spring water, fresh fruit juice, fresh vegetable juice, soup, herbal tea, plant-based milk.

- Cooked foods include a wide variety of vegetables, including legumes and whole grains.

- Plant-based carbohydrates include green leafy vegetables, beans of all kinds, ground provisions, fruits, and whole grains.

- Cooked foods include a wide variety of vegetables, including legumes and whole grains. Avoid overcooking retain as much of the food's nutrients as possible. Vegetables should retain some of their "crunch" or firmness after cooking.

- Plant-based carbohydrates include green leafy vegetables, beans of all kinds, ground provisions, fruits, and whole grains.

- Vegetable sources of protein include various legumes, nuts, seeds, and sea vegetables.

- Vegetable sources of fats include fatty fruits such as avocado and coconut, unrefined nut and seed oils, nut butter, and various nuts and seeds.

Phase III: Live Foods Vegan

The live-foods vegan consumes a plant-based diet of 100% live (uncooked), unprocessed foods. Foods that are uncooked, sun-cooked or heated to no more than 118°F are considered "live." Live foods provide the highest nutritional content and benefits for the body because it is in its purest form. To begin, aim for an intake of live foods at 50% of meals during the winter months, 60-80% of meals during the spring and fall, and 70-100% of meals during the summer months. You may progress toward living a fully raw, live-food diet year-round.

Meal Guidelines:

- Live foods 70-100% of intake

- Cooked foods <30% food

- Live foods include a variety of live fruit and vegetables, soaked nuts and seeds. Live liquids include natural spring water, fresh fruit juice, fresh vegetable juice, sun-fired soups and herbal teas, and plant-based milk.

- Plant-based carbohydrates include green leafy vegetables, sprouted or soaked beans, cooked beans of all kinds, ground provisions, fruits, and whole grains.

- Vegetable sources of protein include sea vegetables and various legumes, nuts, and seeds prepared by soaking and sprouting.

- Vegetable sources of fats include fatty fruits such as avocado and coconut, unrefined nut and seed oils, nut butter, and various nuts and seeds.

- Live foods may be eaten warm to aid digestion. Eating cold foods may cause stomach cramping or aggravate painful menstruation in women. Live foods may be heated to 118° F.

Phase IV: Juicetarian

For detoxing purposes, you may want to spend a specific time nourishing the body with liquid meals. Live foods in liquid form are packed with nutrients and absorbed into the bloodstream quickly. You can accelerate your wellness goals with live fruit and vegetable juices, smoothies, soups, natural spring water and herbal teas.   You may choose to limit the mixing of too many fruits and vegetables at once. Single-ingredient juices are best. Avoid commercial pasteurized juices. Juice should always be made fresh and consumed immediately. Vegetable and fruit juices without the fiber are highly concentrated. This can overwhelm the kidneys or cause the kind of blood sugar spikes that lead to diabetes. For the maximum health benefit, you may dilute juices with 25% to 75% water.

Meal Guidelines:

- Live liquids 100% of intake

- Live liquids include natural spring water, fresh fruit juice, fresh vegetable juice, sun-fired soups and herbal teas, and plant-based milk.

- Single juice ingredients are best for digestion.

- For maximum health benefit, you may dilute juices with 25% to 75% water.

- Juicetarain diet is temporary. Only for specific periods of time for cleansing/detoxing purposes. This detox period generally lasts 7, 14 or 21 days, although some may choose to juice cleanse for as long as 40 days.

Four Levels of Wellness

You are a Divine spiritual being having a Divine human experience. It is important to understand all of the aspects of healing that affect your entire being. A holistic approach to wellness addresses the spiritual, emotional, mental and physical aspects of yourself that create a sense of wholeness and completeness. Every ailment and disease is a manifestation of the mental, emotional and spiritual realm. An imbalance in any of these areas can create imbalances in the others. You may use this concise list to identify any areas of imbalance that are present in your life. Commit to using the suggested healing tools to create a more balanced, healthy lifestyle. From an ancient African and naturopathic perspective, the healing of the disease lies in targeting the disease at its source. In the ancient way, there was no focus on the symptoms. In nurturing the individual with water, food, herbs and spiritual realignment, the person healed themselves.

The Spirit

One having trouble letting go of things in life is suffering from a spiritual disease. Change is the only universal constant inevitable. A part of spiritual maturity comes with being able to flow with the processes of change. Religious fanaticism is a spiritual disease. All disease first exists in the spiritual realm before it manifests in the mind, body and emotions. When it is not dealt with in its unseen form, it comes to the surface in a tangible form to allow us to be able to heal from it. Spiritually differs from religion. To know spiritual balance through universal law is the only truth that has a foundation in the relationship between man and the divine. Religion is defined as a set of beliefs about the existence, nature and worship of deity or deities and divine involvement in the universe and human life. There is no one right religion; they are all opinions and beliefs.

Manifestations of Spiritual Dis-ease

- Doubt or denial of the spiritual reality
- Religious extremism
- Self-consciousness
- Hopelessness
- Lack of faith or belief
- Feeling abandoned by the Most High Creator
- Asking "Why is this happening to me?" in the face of difficulty

- Psychic misinterpretations
- Nightmares
- Insomnia
- Sleep disorders
- Poor memory
- Delusional thinking
- Psychic disturbance

Create a medicine wheel. A medicine wheel, sometimes known as the Sacred Hoop, has been used by generations of Native Americans as a tool for health and healing. It embodies the Four Directions, as well as Father Sky, Mother Earth, and Spirit Tree—all of which symbolize dimensions of health and the cycles of life.

Crystal therapy can be administered by a therapist or self-administered via crystal elixirs, amulets, points of focus, or worn close to the body as jewelry. A crystal is a solid structure composed of molecules that are naturally coordinated, balanced and synchronized with each other. Crystals are not only used in our present-day electronics such as computers, watches and cell phones; they are have been used in ancient times as far back as the first African civilizations to dissipate the negative energies surrounding a person.

RaSekhi Kemetic Reiki is the art form of energetic healing that works through the auric field to clear stagnated energy and raise one's vibration. The "laying on of hands" is an ancient African practice that has been used for relieving stress, melancholy and clearing away traumatic energy that has attached itself to the spiritual body. Through the use of focused awareness and concentration, symbols, hekau (mantras), crystals, aromatherapy, sound and guided meditation RaSekhi can begin to restore balance and harmony within one's entire being.

Prayer is deliberate communication with an object of worship, such as a deity or revered ancestor. It is a devout petition directed at a spiritual source in worship, supplication, gratitude, adoration or confession. Through this invocation of words, one can develop and sustain a relationship with a spiritual source to gain or maintain spiritual power and sustenance.

Meditation is the practice of quiet stillness and focused awareness on a particular thought, object or activity to achieve a calm and stable state of being. During meditation, one is able to develop self-awareness of one's thoughts and emotions without engaging in them. The practice of meditation can instill discipline, clear thinking, self-control and a connection with one's higher consciousness.

Sacred chanting is one of the most ancient spiritual practices wherein high vibrational words or phrases are repeated over and over for the purpose of creating a higher frequency of thinking and behavior. Repetition of the same thought or behavior develops into a habit, which repeated frequently enough, becomes an automatic reflex.

Sound baths and other forms of ***music therapy*** are used to promote healing in all aspects of life through relaxation, the coordination of fine and gross motor skills, motivation and enlightenment. A wide array of instruments are used in music therapy, including piano, chimes, gongs, music bowls, sistrums, rain sticks, clarinets, flutes, tuning forks, drums, tambourines as well as various styles of music. The musical tones target specific organs and areas of the body. Higher notes, as in flutes and classical music, stimulate the brain, neurological functions, communication and spiritual development.

The middle range notes in soul, reggae and hip-hop music affect the midsection, including the heart, lungs, stomach and all thoracic organs. Lower tones created by the bass and drums stimulate the sexual organs and lower extremities.

Draw a mandala. A mandala is a geometric figure used in Indo-Asian religions like Hinduism and Buddhism to represent the universe. It is a cosmic diagram, used as an instrument in meditation, which symbolizes completeness and unity.

Start a vision board. A vision board is a collage of images and words used as a visual tool to help you manifest your goals and desires through the law of attraction. A vision board is a creative process to set clear intentions for what you want in life so you can grow and transform yourself.

Sun bathing is the simple act of sitting or laying in the sun. The sun is the center of our solar system, powering every living thing in existence on the earth and every plant in the known universe. Exposure to the sun not only increases your body's levels of Vitamin D, but it has also been proven to boost mood, feelings of relaxation and creativity.

Spend time in nature. As human beings living in a modern world of technology, we often forget that we are, in fact, a part of nature. The further and further we get from nature, the sicker we become. Spending time in nature reminds us of our connectedness to the totality of all existence.

Keep a dream journal. The dream world is the dimension where our subconscious mind works through the events of daily living. The symbols we receive in dreams are visual messages that we can interpret for guidance and develop stronger intuition in our waking lives. You may want to keep a dream journal and a pen close to your bed. Write down your dream as soon as possible after waking, as the messages are often lost from memory as you awaken. You can use a dream dictionary to interpret specific symbols and uncover the deeper meaning of the dreams.

Take a spiritual bath. This is a ritual bath that cleanses the chakras and revitalizes the auric field. This can be helpful in times of stress or trauma to uplift and strengthen the spirit. It can also be used to assist in manifesting specific desires or goals. Spiritual bath tools include herbs, crystals, candles, flowers, specific food items, and essential oils and fragrances added to the bath water. Prayers, mantras, or affirmations are often spoken to program the water molecules to your desired intentions.

Create an altar. An altar is a sacred space used to honor your spiritual source or revered ancestors. You may use this as a peaceful space to gain clarity and wisdom on your wellness journey and daily life. Altar work may include prayer, meditation, affirmations, music, chanting, incense and offering specific food items such as wine, fruit and honey. Your altar can help you to stay connected to the intentions you set for your life.

Manifestations of Spiritual Wellness

- Feeling connected to your spiritual source
- Being in this world but not of this world
- Able to spend quiet time alone just being
- Integration
- The experience of all as one
- Joy and peace
- Trusting in the Most High
- Asking what can be learned from difficulty
- Intuitiveness
- Clairvoyance
- Clairaudience
- Clairsentience,
- Self-actualization
- Virtuousness

The Mind

The mind is the most powerful tool we have in creating our reality. You literally are what you think you are. Stress, abuse or trauma, especially when experienced early in life, can trigger negative thought patterns that create a matching reality. Persistent thoughts of unworthiness, guilt, shame, rejection, abandonment, and loneliness set up an emotional tailspin that takes a person further off the path of self-actualization. As these negative thought patterns lead a person down any number of dysfunctional avenues in life, it can become more difficult to recognize these negative thoughts for the delusions that they are. Delusions are thoughts and thought patterns that are out of alignment with what is real, true and factual. Despite whatever problems these delusions have created in a person's life, we each have the power to restructure the brain and manifest a whole new reality.

Manifestations of Mental Dis-ease

- Cunning, deceit without lying or creative lying
- Shyness
- Speaking too bluntly
- Fear
- Panic and overwhelm
- Neurosis
- Obsessive or addictive behavior
- Drug and alcohol abuse
- Suicidal thinking
- Boredom
- Impatience
- Inability to focus on one thing
- Denial of actual experiences in reality
- Confusion of what is real and what appears real
- Being "out of it," out of the body or out of touch with the body

- Rigid conformity

- Closed-mindedness

- Racism

- Projection

- Blame

- Psychosis

- Hyper-intellectuality to withdraw from emotions

- Greed

Healing Tools

Journaling is the act of writing to help you prioritize, clarify thinking and accomplish important tasks. The act of daily or frequent or daily journaling can be a life-changing habit. Journaling encourages clear communication and expression of oneself and can lead to honest communication in relationships with others.

Cognitive-behavioral therapy is a psycho-social intervention that aims to improve mental health. A licensed therapist focuses on challenging and changing unhelpful thought patterns and behaviors, improving emotional regulation and developing personal coping strategies that target solving current problems.

Writing and reciting poetry is a form of literary expression that improves writing skills and vocabulary and encourages creative thinking. Reciting poetry opens up the throat chakra for clearer communication, pitch, rhythm, tone and sound of voice.

Affirmations are positive statements or declarations that can help you to overcome self-sabotaging, negative thinking and behaviors. Every thought creates a biochemical reaction in the brain that sends a signal or instruction to the rest of the body. It is inferred then that positive affirmations can be used to alter the biochemistry of the brain and are quite powerful tools for healing.

Singing can have a soothing, yet energizing effect on one's entire being. Singing is a natural anti-depressant that improves confidence, lowers stress levels and improves mental alertness. It also aids in opening the throat chakra for more inspirational communication.

Breath therapy is the application of specific breathing techniques to induce healing states within the mind, body and spirit. The conscious process of breath control work can assist in recovering from lower mental states such as fear, panic and depression.

Practicing mindfulness is the therapeutic process of focusing one's awareness on the present moment while calming, acknowledging and accepting one's feelings, thoughts, and bodily sensations. Mindfulness is a powerful tool for achieving self-awareness, self-realization, clear perception and being in the present moment.

Stargazing is the simple act of observing the stars. It is often done in natural environments or high up on a hill or mountain where the view is not obstructed by pollution or tall buildings. Stargazing fosters feelings of expansion, inspiration, imagination, alleviates stress and increases happiness.

Crossword puzzles are a form of word search games that involve solving clues that lead to the answers. They can be quite beneficial in releasing stress, improving vocabulary, memory, mental health and brain function.

Color therapy, or chromotherapy, is a natural remedy that uses color and light to address physical or mental health imbalances, including anger, melancholy blood pressure, learning disabilities, insomnia and academic performance. This practice dates back to ancient Kemet, where sun-activated solarium rooms with colored glass were used for therapeutic purposes. Each color produces certain effects on the mind, emotions, energy level, mood and behavior.

Learning a new language can increase confidence, as mastering any new skill does. It sharpens the mind, improves memory and multi-tasking abilities, and enhances decision making. Language is also the best expression of a culture. In healing through your cultural practices, language can be a powerful tool.

Self-reflection is the process of introspection and serious thought about one's own character, actions and motives. It is one's attempt to learn more about one's fundamental nature and essence. This form of self-observation and analysis allows a person to grow in wisdom and develop accountability for one's own actions.

Manifestations of Mental Wellness

- Honesty
- Ability to think and express yourself clearly
- Inspirational communication
- Confidence
- Being listened to as an authoritative voice
- Direct knowing
- Self-possession
- Passion for life
- Diligence
- Self-realization
- Self-determination
- Self-awareness
- Clear perception
- Being in the present moment
- Creativity
- Open to new ideas without being naive
- Expansion
- Discovery and exploration
- Accountable for one's own actions
- Wisdom
- Service to others

The Emotions

An excess amount of emotional outpour of any kind- anger, sadness, joy, confusion, grief, fear is an indication of emotional disease. Meant to help us learn from our environment. When we dwell on the negative feeling of it, we create and internal cesspool of emotional debris that will wreak havoc in all areas of their life. This manifestation is a result of the person consistently not internalizing the lesson(s) of the emotion.

Manifestations of Emotional Dis-ease

- Unhealthy forms of attachment
- Despair
- Loneliness
- Alienation
- Need for external validation

- Passive aggression
- Avoidance of intimacy
- Consideration of oneself regardless of others
- Distrustful or hostile relationship to the world

ABRAHAM HICKS EMOTIONAL GUIDANCE SCALE

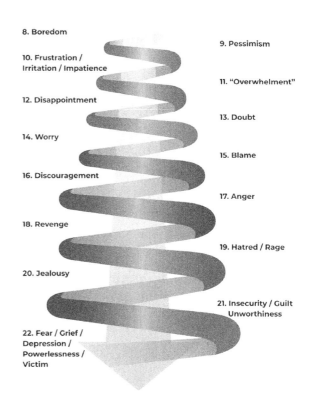

UPWARD SPIRAL

1. Joy/ Knowledge empowerment freedom / Love Appreciation
2. Passion
3. Enthusiasm
4. Positive Expectation Belief
5. Optimism
6. Hopefulness
7. Contentment

DOWNWARD SPIRAL

8. Boredom
9. Pessimism
10. Frustration / Irritation / Impatience
11. "Overwhelment"
12. Disappointment
13. Doubt
14. Worry
15. Blame
16. Discouragement
17. Anger
18. Revenge
19. Hatred / Rage
20. Jealousy
21. Insecurity / Guilt Unworthiness
22. Fear / Grief / Depression / Powerlessness / Victim

- Workaholism driven by a lack of self-worth
- Hatred
- Questioning the existence of love
- Rage
- Lack of boundaries in relationships
- Guilt
- Self-shaming
- Shame
- Perpetual victimhood
- Apathy

Emotional Healing Tools

Cultivating and practicing self-love simply means to have high regard for your own well-being and happiness. It is not an act of selfishness, although this concept can be difficult to grasp for those who have developed the habit of people-pleasing. Self-love means prioritizing your own needs above pleasing others and not accepting less than what you desire.

Art therapy is a visual form of expressive therapy that assists people to resolve issues, reduce stress, improve self-esteem and awareness, and manage their behaviors and feelings. It can include painting or drawing with various supplies either alone or with a group under the guidance of an art therapist. It is a very effective treatment for persons experiencing psychological or emotional stress.

Walking in moonlight is an effective, natural way to reduce stress and improve mood by increasing levels of vitamin D and endorphins. Just as the moon affects the tides of the oceans, it also affects the waters within the body's systems. Regular exposure to moonlight may also aid in regulating menstrual cycles for women.

Spend time with supportive family or friends is an essential factor in creating strong bonds, love, connections and relationships. It is important for those who may have experienced dysfunctional or toxic family relationships to discover and create those supportive relationships with other family members or friends. Healthy, harmonious relationships with others is fundamental to cultivating our own human development.

Forgiveness is a conscious, deliberate decision to release feelings of anger, resentment and vengeance toward someone who has harmed you. Holding onto the anger of actual or perceived injustice is like drinking poison and expecting the other person to die. The act of forgiveness can free you from anger and bitterness that will inevitably destroy your peace and happiness. Forgiveness is not simply letting go of resentment. To forgive, you must give or extend yourself in some way to the person who has harmed you. Essentially, it is a gift given to the other person that you reap the ultimate reward from.

Visiting natural environments such as parks, beaches, rivers, waterfalls, and mountains is a great way to hit the emotional reset button. Connecting to nature is a powerful healing tool for neutralizing low vibration emotional states like boredom, worry, grief and depression and anger. The negative ions generated by the natural atmosphere neutralizes free-radicals, revitalizes cell metabolism and produces a euphoric emotional state.

A reiki circle is a small group of healers who gather together to practice reiki healing modalities to promote energetic, emotional and physical well-being. Group healing amplifies and enhances the energy of reiki. Within a group session, healers are able to concentrate and direct a group's healing energy.

Gratitude is the feeling or act of thankfulness and appreciation, which is highest on the vibrational scale of emotions. Practicing the expression of gratitude is one of the quickest and most effective ways to raise your vibrational frequency.

Emotional Freedom Technique (EFT), or tapping, is a holistic treatment for physical pain and emotional distress. It is a form of counseling intervention that draws on various natural therapies such as acupuncture, neurolinguistic programming, energy medicine and Thought-Field therapy. Without needles, an EFT therapist will use the fingertips to tap on emotional energy points to assist the client in releasing blockages in these areas.

Mirror work is a therapeutic form of confidence-building in which you meet your reflection in the mirror to open up a conversation with yourself as if you are speaking with a dear friend. During mirror work sessions, you practice speaking loving, self-affirming statements to yourself for the purpose of self-discovery and developing a deeper level of unconditional self-love.

Practice self-awareness. This is the ability to see yourself clearly through the process of introspection and self-reflection. It is through the practice of self-awareness that we can clearly perceive our own values, passions, aspirations and develop a greater degree of emotional control.

Assertiveness training is a learned mode of communication based on the principle that we have a right to express our thoughts, feelings and needs to others as long as we do so in a respectful way. This is a helpful tool for those who are people pleasers or have difficulty creating healthy boundaries with others.

Shadow work is the process of unveiling and becoming aware of the hidden aspects of oneself that may be viewed by the ego as shameful or unworthy. This can be done alone or under the guidance of a trained healer or therapist. Shadow work encourages compassion, freedom from judgment and unconditional self-love. When working with the shadow self, you may have moments of awakening that lead to greater fulfillment, authenticity and emotional freedom.

Volunteering to charitable causes is a benefit to others and also to yourself. Volunteering combats loneliness, increases socializing, builds bonds, creates friends, builds community, and provides a sense of purpose. Altruistic activities promote unconditional love for all, a sense of internal power, and empathy.

Cultivate your talents and skills. It is virtually impossible to feel a sense of purpose, confidence or self-esteem without cultivating your divinely given talents and skills. Each of us has a set of talents that the world needs. Our skills and talents are not given to us for us, but to contribute to the world.

Manifestations of Emotional Wellness

- Mutually empowering relationships
- Acceptance that all is as it should be
- Valuing oneself
- Sincerity
- Awareness of the effect of one's actions upon others
- Harmonious relationships
- Harmony with nature
- Passion for life

- Genuine intimacy
- Allowing oneself to be vulnerable
- Setting appropriate boundaries
- Self-acceptance
- Control over one's life
- Unconditional love for all
- Empathy
- Will power

The Body

As whole beings, any illness of the spiritual, mental, or emotional bodies can create illness in the physical body. Physical illness is most often created by our lifestyle choices, which are a manifestation of our spiritual, mental and emotional states of being. The physical body must have the proper internal and external environment to facilitate healing. Removing toxic foods and chemicals from the diet while nourishing the body with natural food, water, herbs creates the proper internal environment for wellness. Inner-outer balance occurs when we create a lifestyle that allows us to access the healing power of nature's elements- air, fire, water, earth and ether.

Physical Manifestations of Dis-ease

- Tension
- Stress
- Chronic pain
- Fatigue

- Exhaustion
- Shame of the body or sexuality
- Exhibitionism or over the top displays
- Hyper-sexuality or sexual addiction

- Overweight or underweight
- Disordered eating
- Disease
- Trauma

- Injury
- Loss of function
- Paralysis or coma

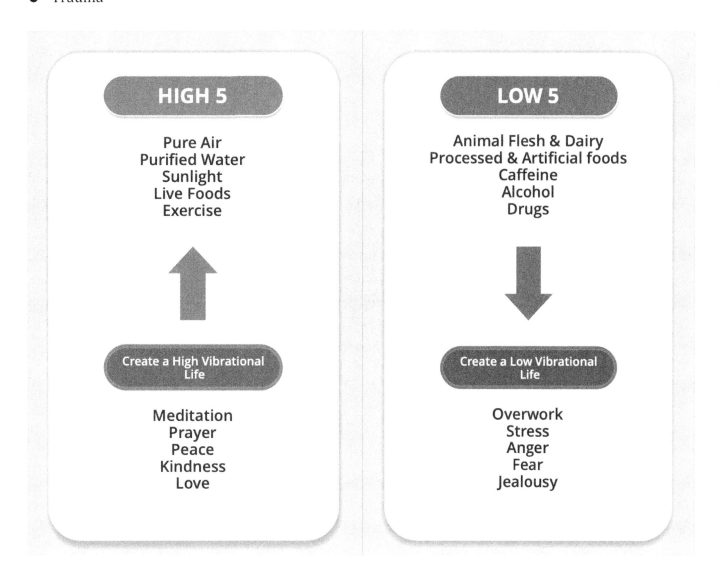

Physical Healing Tools

Rest, the deliberate cease from action or motion, is a necessary component of healing that is often neglected. It is essential for proper human functioning to take periods throughout the day to refrain from exertion to allow for cellular renewal.

Sound sleep is absolutely vital for all aspects of good health. It is important for maintaining energy levels and a strong immune system, lowering stress and blood pressure, regulating weight, and improving memory.

Kemetic sacred movement, also known as Kemetic Yoga, are the postures and positions of the *nTrw* (NETCHERU- divine laws and principles), which open up energy vortexes in the body. This ancient practice emerging from Nile Valley African civilization was used to strengthen the *sekhem* (internal vital power), to still the mind and access one's higher consciousness. Kemetic sacred movement is the origin of today's widely known Indo-Asian yoga forms such as Hatha Yoga, Vinyasa Yoga and Kundalini Yoga.

Physical exercise in any number of forms, including walking, running, biking, has innumerable benefits for the body and the mind. Exercise is a great tool for weight management, lowering blood pressure, and increasing blood sugar control. The chemical endorphins released after exercise greatly improves mental health and mood.

Pilates is an exercise system developed in the 1920s by German physical trainer Joseph Hubertus Pilates. It is a low-impact form of exercise that combines muscle strengthening with flexibility and proper postural alignment. Regular practice of Pilates can improve muscle control, balance, strength and flexibility.

Martial arts, including boxing, judo, karate and kung fu is an excellent form of cardiovascular exercise. Some African martial forms include Dambe, Kupigana Ngumi, Laamb, Tahtib and Capoeira. The practice of martial arts improves focus, discipline and stillness. There is a code of conduct within various martial arts systems that teaches morals and values. Personal development in the area of self-defense increases self-confidence, self-mastery, and athleticism.

Dancing is an excellent way to release toxins and negative energy that have been stored in the body's tissues. Cultural dance has the added benefit of increasing a sense of self-empowerment, connectedness and self-esteem. The fluid movements in dancing can assist in healing imbalances related to sexuality, negative body image and sexual trauma.

Swimming and water aerobics are forms of aquatic exercise that can aid mobility and joint flexibility, increase lung capacity and cardiovascular strength with very low impact on the joints.   Swimming is also an excellent way to tone muscles, build strength and endurance and maintain a healthy weight.

Saunas are small rooms that are a source of dry heat with temperatures ranging between 150º F and 195º F . Sauna rooms are often made of unpainted wood. The high temperatures help the blood vessels to relax, increasing blood circulation, reducing muscle and joint tension, and relieving chronic pain and stress. The heat also cleanses the body as toxins are released from the skin through sweating.

A whirlpool is a body of rotating water created by the meeting of opposing currents. Sitting in a whirlpool for regular 20 minute periods can benefit those with joint inflammation issues such as Carpal Tunnel Syndrome, Fibromyalgia, Tendonitis, Scoliosis and Bursitis.

Steam bathing with essential oils is a form of hydrotherapy that can be performed as a regular part of your self-care routine. It is an excellent form of stress-relief and a highly effective mood booster. The fragrance of the essential oils also gives off the added benefits of aromatherapy. The warm water allows the essential oils to penetrate the skin while the scent of the oils is inhaled at the same time.

Massage is a therapeutic form of touch involving the rubbing and kneading of the body's muscles and joints, usually to relieve tension or pain. This can be performed by a licensed therapist or a close friend or family member. However, self-massage is also quite beneficial when receiving a professional massage is not possible. The stimulation of the nerve endings promotes relaxation, good circulation and the elimination of stagnant energy.

Reflexology is an ancient natural massage therapy used to alleviate tension and release stagnant energy in the lymphatic, circulatory and nervous systems. A certified reflexologist uses specific massage techniques on the hands, feet and head to stimulate the receptors linked to every part of the body. When done consistently, reflexology can enhance the body's ability to metabolize nutrients, increase energy and mood levels, and aid in proper blood circulation to all organ systems.

Foot soaks are beneficial for soothing sore muscles, hydrating dry skin and relieving pain from standing or walking for long hours or walking in uncomfortable shoes. Different types of foot soaks have different benefits. A 10-minute foot bath in ice water can reduce the swelling of walking in high heels. Soaking the feet in a warm Epsom salt bath has the added benefits of relieving muscle soreness, preventing toenail fungus, and inhibiting the growth of bacteria in open sores or blisters.

Plant-based nutrition is essentially a vegetarian dietary regimen in which animal products are eliminated or strictly limited. Those who enjoy a plant-based lifestyle often report relief of constipation due to the increase in dietary fiber. Many people also transition to a plant-based diet to increase nutrients in the body for the purpose of weight management and to eliminate or prevent dis-ease.

Colon irrigation or colon hydrotherapy is the process of flushing the colon with large amounts of water to remove excess waste. This therapy is done under the care of a trained, certified therapist. Regular colon cleansing is also a form of self-care which can be done via enema or with the use of herbs such as senna or cascara sagrada.

Calisthenics is a form of resistance training using your own bodyweight. This form of muscle training can create a leaner muscular appearance without the added stress from dumbbells or weight machines. Popular calisthenic exercises include planks, sits, pull-ups, handstands and burpees. Regular calisthenic exercise can improve strength.

Herbal therapy is the use of plants for their medicinal and healing properties. The herbs of the land are for the healing of the nations. The term "alternative therapy" applied to herbal medicine is quite a misnomer, as herbalism is the most ancient form of medicine. In fact, over 70% of modern pharmaceuticals are derived from plants.

Chiropractic care is the practice of adjusting or manipulating the spine to correct alignment problems, ease pain and support the body's natural ability to heal itself. The process is done by a Licensed Chiropractor for the purpose of correcting disorders o the musculoskeletal and nervous systems and the effects thereof. Emphasizes the body's ability to heal itself. Used to restore mobility to joints restricted by tissue injury caused by a traumatic event, such as falling or repetitive stress, such as sitting without proper back support. Chiropractic treatment is primarily used as a pain relief alternative for muscles, joints, bones, and connective tissue, such as cartilage, ligaments, and tendons.

Acupressure an alternative medicine technique, is similar in principle to acupuncture. It is based on the concept of life energy, which flows through meridians in the body. In treatment, physical pressure is applied to acupuncture points with the aim of clearing blockages in these meridians. In treatment, physical pressure is applied to acupuncture points with the aim of clearing blockages in these meridians.

Acupuncture is a form of treatment that involves inserting very thin needles through a person's skin at specific points on the body to various depths. Research suggests that it can help relieve pain, and it is used for a wide range of other complaints. It is a 3,000 year-old healing technique of Traditional Chinese Medicine. Acupuncture seeks to release the flow of the body's vital energy or "*chi*" by stimulating points along 14 energy pathways. Some scientists believe that the needles cause the body to release endorphins -- natural painkillers -- and may boost blood flow and change brain activity.

Physical therapy aims to ease pain and help you function, move, and live better. It is facilitated by a licensed Physical Therapist to relieve pain and improve movement or ability, Prevent or recover from an injury, Prevent disability or surgery, Rehab after a stroke, accident, injury, or surgery, Work on balance to prevent a slip or fall, Learn to use an assistive device like a walker or cane.

Manifestations of Physical Wellness

- Flexibility
- Comfort
- Ease
- Physical energy
- Stamina
- Strength

- Being comfortable in your body and sexuality
- Having a healthy relationship with food
- Perfect health
- Physically healthy and active
- Joyful movement
- Full presence

21-Day Detox

Begin your transition to plant-based eating with a 21-day detox. During your detox, you will eliminate 1. Processed, microwave and artificial GMO food 2. Animal Flesh 3. Dairy 4. Coffee 5. Alcohol. This will allow you to cleanse the body of low vibration foods. One of the most effective ways to begin a new habit or break an old one is to incorporate a new change for 21 days. Learn from any slip-ups or challenges you may have and move forward toward your goal. Every single meal is another opportunity to start fresh. The key is consistency, not perfection. You may choose to detox yearly, biannually or seasonally, depending on your personal wellness goals. You may continue to track your progress throughout the next 6 months of your wellness journey.

Track Your Progress

Start date: _____   Start weight: _____

Goal Weight: _____   Date achieved: _____

WEEK	DATE	CURRENT WEIGHT	WEEK	DATE	CURRENT WEIGHT
1			15		
2			16		
3			17		
4			18		
5			19		
6			20		
7			21		
8			22		
9			23		
10			24		
11			25		
12			26		
13			27		
14			28		

Wellness Goals

Most people have at least 5 health challenges. Take a minute to assess what health challenges you may be experiencing and decide on the goals you want to achieve to live your best life. Be sure to include a target date for when you desire to accomplish your goals.

What are your current health challenges?

What are your wellness goals?

Obstacles to achieving my goals:

Action steps to achieving your wellness goals:

How will I benefit from achieving my goals?

How will my family and community benefit from me achieving my goals?

Date	Health Challenge	Wellness Goal	Target Date	Date Resolved

21 Days of
Self-Reflection

Begin each day with *heka / hekau* (words of power). These words are taken from the *mdw ntchr* [medew netcher], the ancient language of the African Nile Valley Civilization commonly known as hieroglyphs. This language, which literally means Divine words of The Creator, encourages self-love and empowerment for a healthy, prosperous life. Positive affirmations modify thought patterns and counteract negative thoughts. Daily journal writing facilitates awareness to improve mental and emotional wellness.

Day 1

Heka:

skhm [sekhem]- internal vital power

Affirmation:

I am healthy and full of energy.

Journal:

Draw a picture of yourself happy, healthy and whole.

Day 2

Heka:

nfr [nefer]- beautiful

Affirmation:

The universe helps me achieve beautiful levels of health and wellness.

Journal:

Name three things you accomplished today.

Day 3

Heka:

diw [diu]- gift

Affirmation:

My body is the most precious gift.

Journal:

What made you smile today?

Day 4

Heka:

maat [MA'AT] - balance, harmony

Affirmation:

I am balanced- mind, body, and spirit.

Journal:

What do you wish there was less of in the world?

Day 5

Heka:

rxt [rekhet] (knowledge)

Affirmation:

All of my cells know exactly what to do.

Journal:

Who inspires you? Why?

Day 6

Heka:

rhn [rhen]- to trust

Affirmation:

I trust my body.

Journal:

Am I using my strengths often enough?

Day 7

Heka:

mr [mer]- to love

Affirmation:

I choose health, happiness, and love for myself and others.

Journal:

What was the last thing that made you laugh out loud?

Day 8

Heka:

rnpy [renpy]- to be young, fresh, vigorous, healthy

Affirmation:

Everything I eat and drink heals me.

Journal:

What motivated you today?

Day 9

Heka:

snb [seneb]- health

Affirmation:

My healthy body reflects my healthy thoughts and feelings.

Journal:

What are you most grateful for?

Day 10

Heka:

rwD [rudj]- strength

Affirmation:

I am filled with strength and vitality.

Journal:

Who is the last person to tell you they love you?

Day 11

Heka:

Ssp [shesep]- to accept

Affirmation:

I fully accept where I am, and I seize this opportunity to grow.

Journal:

I could be more productive if I stopped...

Day 12

Heka:

xnty snb [khenty seneb]- picture of health

Affirmation:

I am the picture of positivity and well-being.

Journal:

What made today unusual?

Day 13

Heka:

tiw [tiu]- yes

Affirmation:

As I say yes to life, life says yes to me.

Journal:

The best part of today was

Day 14

Heka:

nTr [NETCHER]- The Divine One Most High Creator

Affirmation:

The divine healing power of the universe flows through my mind, body and spirit.

Journal:

Describe a challenging situation you had this week and how you overcame it.

Day 15

Heka

mwt [mut]- mother

Affirmation:

I tend to my body with unconditional love and care.

Journal:

Some things I can do to experience more joy in my life are...

Day 16

Heka:

anx [ankh]- life

Affirmation:

I release all resistance to a healthful life. A life of wellness is mine now.

Journal:

What is your purpose?

Day 17

Heka

anuk - I am

Affirmation:

I accept and love myself just the way I am.

Journal:

What does a good day look like for you?

Day 18

Heka:

tm [tem]- to be complete, be whole, be perfect

Affirmation:

I am grateful that I am happy, whole and healthy.

Journal:

Is my health harming my purpose in life?

Day 19

Heka

wp [wep]- to open

Affirmation:

I am open to new ways of improving my health.

Journal:

What would I do if I had six months to live?

Day 20

Heka:

HAty [haty]- desire

Affirmation:

I am a magnet for positive energy and good health.

Journal:

Name three good habits you want to adopt this year.

Day 21

Heka:

rk [rek]- time

Affirmation:

I deserve the best, and I accept it now.

Journal:

Dear Future Me...

Kitchen Tools

- Baking sheets
- Baking tins
- Biodegradable dishwashing soap
- Blender
- Can opener
- Ceramic mugs
- Cheese cloth
- Citrus juicer
- Cork screw
- Decorative dishes
- Dehydrator
- Foil
- Food processor
- Funnels
- Garbage bags
- Glassware
- Grater
- Hand mixer
- Juicer
- Kitchen shears
- Mason Jars (various sizes)
- Measuring cups
- Measuring spoons
- Mortar and pestle
- Oven gloves
- Parchment paper
- Paper towels
- Potato masher

- Pressure cooker
- Recycle bags
- Rolling pins
- Salad spinner
- Serving trays
- Serving utensils
- Slow cooker
- Spiralizer
- Stainless steel/cast iron/enamel pots and pans
- Strainer
- Table cloths
- Tea kettle
- Tongs
- Vegan recipe books
- Vegetable slicer
- Vegetable scrubber
- Vegetable wash
- Wheatgrass juicer
- Whisk
- Wood cutting boards

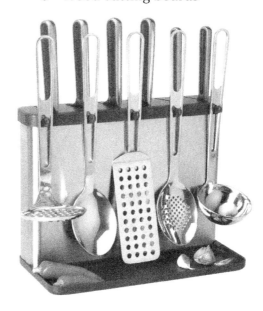

High Vibration Food Shopping List

Vegetables (And fruits eaten as vegetables)

- Ackee
- Artichoke
- Asparagus
- Avocado
- Beets
- Broccoli
- Bokchoy
- Cabbage
- Cassava
- Cauliflower
- Celery
- Carrots
- Cucumber
- Dandelion greens
- Dill
- Eggplant
- Green banana
- Irish moss/ sea moss
- Kale
- Kelp
- Leeks
- Mixed greens
- Onions
- Radishes
- Romaine lettuce
- Parsley
- Peppers
- Plantain
- Spinach
- Squash
- Sugar snap peas
- Sweet potato
- Swiss chard
- Tomato
- Turnips
- Wheatgrass
- Yam
- Zucchini

Fruit

- Apples
- Banana
- Blueberry
- Cantaloupe
- Cherry
- Cranberry
- Coconut
- Dates
- Figs
- Grapes
- Grapefruit
- Guava
- Honey dew
- Jackfruit
- Kiwi
- Lemon/lime
- Lychee
- Mango
- Orange
- Papaya
- Peach
- Pear
- Persimmon
- Plums
- Prunes
- Pineapple
- Pomegranates
- Raisins
- Raspberry
- Watermelon

Whole grains

- Amaranth
- Barley
- Brown rice
- Bulgar
- Buckwheat
- Corn
- Couscous
- Millet
- Oat
- Quinoa
- Rye
- Spelt
- Wheat germ
- Whole grain flour
- Whole grain spelt bread
- Whole grain waffles
- Whole grain pasta

Legumes (beans, nuts, seeds and sprouts)

- Alfalfa sprouts
- Almonds
- Black beans
- Black-eyed peas
- Cannelloni beans
- Cashews
- Chia seeds
- Chickpeas
- Flaxseeds
- Kidney beans
- Hazelnuts
- Lentils
- Lima beans
- Macadamias
- Mung bean sprouts

- Pinto beans
- Pistachios
- Pumpkin seeds
- Sunflower seeds
- Walnuts
- Oils and butters
- Almond butter
- Almond oil
- Castor oil
- Coconut oil
- Cold pressed olive oil
- Grapeseed oil
- Peanut butter
- Sesame oil
- Sunflower oil
- Vegan butter spread
- Vegan mayonaise

Liquids:

- Almond milk
- Black tea
- Coconut milk
- Coconut water
- Hazelnut milk
- Herbal tea
- Hemp milk
- Oat milk
- Organic apple juice
- Organic orange juice
- Purified water
- Rice milk
- Vegetable soups

Sweeteners:

- Agave
- Cane sugar
- Maple syrup
- Molasses

- Raw honey
- Stevia leaf

Miscellaneous:

- Apple cider
- Vinegar
- Beet powder
- Bee pollen
- Chlorella powder
- Garlic kyolic
- Liquid aminos
- Nutritional yeast
- Spirulina powder
- Wheatgrass powder

Herbs & spices:

- Alfafa
- Basil
- Cayenne pepper
- Cascara sagrada
- Chamomile
- Cinnamon
- Citrus peel
- Cloves
- Coriander
- Cumin
- Curry
- Dandelion
- Dill
- Fennel
- Fenugreek
- Garlic
- Ginger
- Goldenseal
- Hibiscus
- Lemongrass
- Moringa
- Neem

- Nutmeg
- Oregano
- Paprika
- Parsley
- Rosemary
- Peppermint
- Red raspberry
- Cooking sage
- Sea salt
- Spearmint
- Sun dried tomato
- Tomato sauce
- Tomato paste
- Turmeric
- Thyme
- Valerian

Environmentally friendly household items:

- Trash bags
- Blue recycle bags
- Biodegradable dish soap
- Biodegradable laundry detergent
- Household cleaner
- Paper towels
- Toilet paper

Other:

- —
- —
- —
- —
- —
- —
- —
- —

High Vibration
Meal Plan

7 Days of High Vibration Vegetarian Nutrition

Sunday	Monday	Tuesday	Wednesday	Thursday	Friday	Saturday
Breakfast	**Breakfast**	**Breakfast**	**Breakfast**	**Breakfast**	**Breakfast**	**Breakfast**
Herbal tea 1-2 Sliced honey crisp apples Oatmeal Casserole	Herbal tea Fresh mango Juice Tropical Fruit Platter	Herbal tea Papaya, banana smoothie. Avocado on sprouted toast	Berry Juice Smoothie Nutty cinnamon quinoa hot cereal	1 cup strawberries (or fruit of choice). Green banana porridge	Warm lemon water 1 cup mixed berries. Vegan blueberry waffles	Carrot Juice Caribbean Big Breakfast.
TIP: Drink water before each meal.	TIP: Single ingredient juices are best for digestion.	TIP: Always break your fast with light foods such as natural juice, tea and fruit.	TIP: Vegetarian meals include 50%-70% live foods.	TIP: You can "veganize" any of your favorite recipes. Be creative!	TIP: Use a vegan egg replacer and almond milk (or plant-based milk of choice)	TIP: Use carrot pulp to make carrot "tuna" for lunch
Lunch	**Lunch**	**Lunch**	**Lunch**	**Lunch**	**Lunch**	**Lunch**
Juice: Kale, apple, lemon Lentil Soup Garden Salad Kale Sandwich	Quinoa veggie burger Creamy Coleslaw Juice: Spinach, cucumber, apple	Juice: Carrot, apple, beet, ginger Creamy Lemon Garlic Alfredo Zucchini Pasta	Juice: Spinach, cucumber, lemon Garden Salad Veggie Pizza	Juice: Kale, apple, lemon Creamy kale salad Tabouli	Mixed greens salad Ital red bean stew Herbal tea	Carrot Juice mixed greens salad Carrot "tuna" over sprouted bread
TIP: For **weight loss/ maintenance**, eat the lightest foods first: (1) Liquids (2) Greens (3) Heavy Starches (4) Protein (5) Fats	TIP: For **weight gain,** eat the heaviest foods first: (1) Fats (2) Proteins (3) Heavy Starches (4) Greens (5) Liquids	TIP: Dilute juice with 25% to 75% water to avoid blood sugar spikes.	TIP: Fruits detoxify the body, which vegetables nourish and repair.	TIP: Live foods may be warmed to room temperature to aid digestion.	TIP: Eat the cultural foods of your ancestors. Your healing is in your culture.	TIP: Drink half your body weight in oz. daily. Ex: 140 lb. woman should consume 70 oz. (8.75 cups) water daily.
Dinner	**Dinner**	**Dinner**	**Dinner**	**Dinner**	**Dinner**	**Dinner**
Avocado Salad Spaghetti with falafel balls in marinara sauce. Herbal tea	Grated apple, beet, carrot, cabbage salad. Sweet plantains Sautéed mushrooms served over couscous Herbal tea	Collard greens Baked breadfruit Jerk jackfruit vegan "pulled chicken" Herbal tea	Mixed Greens Salad Curry chickpeas stuffed sweet potato Herbal tea	Spinach salad Spaghetti with falafel balls in marinara sauce Herbal tea	Dandelion greens salad Steamed asparagus Sautéed Eggplant Cook-Up Herbal tea	Steamed broccoli Mashed Potatoes BBQ Mushroom ribs Herbal tea
TIP: Replace wheat pasta with spiralized zucchini for a gluten-free option.	TIP: Drink hot herbal tea after meals to aid digestion.	TIP: Conclude eating by 7 pm. If hungry after this time, fruit, green juice, tea or soup is best.	TIP: Consider food combining when preparing meals.	TIP: Homemade sauces and dressings are best over store-bought.	TIP: For maximum benefit, steep herbal tea at least 10-15 minutes before drinking.	TIP: Eat a balance of 50-70% live foods and 30-50% steamed/cooked foods.

Create Your Own Menu

Sunday	Monday	Tuesday	Wednesday	Thursday	Friday	Saturday
Breakfast	Breakfast	Breakfast	Breakfast	Breakfast	Breakfast	Breakfast
Lunch	Lunch	Lunch	Lunch	Lunch	Lunch	Lunch
Dinner	Dinner	Dinner	Dinner	Dinner	Dinner	Dinner

High Vibration Recipes

Tip: Single ingredient juices are best for digestion. Vegetable and fruit juices juices without the fiber are highly concentrated. This can overwhelm the kidneys or cause the kind of blood sugar spikes that lead to diabetes. For the maximum health benefit, you may dilute juices with 25% to 75% of water.

Delicious Single Ingredient Juices

- Carrot Juice (eye health)
- Honeydew Melon Juice (bone health)
- Papaya Juice (ease menstrual pain)
- Yam Juice (fertility)
- Pineapple Juice (cold and sinus)
- Watermelon Juice (hydration)
- Pomegranate (heart disease prevention)
- Kiwi (healthy skin)
- Strawberry (lowers blood pressure)
- Beets (prevent anemia)
- Coconut (electrolyte balance)
- Cucumber (reduce bad breath)
- Cranberry (urinary tract health)

- Cauliflower (brain booster)
- Spinach (treats hemophilia)
- Apple (aids digestion)
- Pear (prevent birth defects)
- Blackberry (improve brain function)
- Grapefruit (treats fever)
- Orange (boosts immune system)
- Grape (colon health)
- Mango (treat acne)
- Celery (treats rheumatism)
- String bean (blood sugar control)
- Cabbage (anti-ulcer)

Juicing vs. blending

Juice is extracted using a juicer. The juice of the fruit or vegetable is separated from the fiber. High water content fruits and vegetables are best for juicing.	Juice is made using a high-powered blender. The whole fruit or vegetable is blended into a liquid.

Juice is extracted using a juicer. The juice of the fruit or vegetable is separated from the fiber. High water content fruits and vegetables are best for juicing.

Citrus fruits are best juiced alone or with other citrus fruits. May combine with greens or sub-acid fruits. Extract juice using a citrus juicer for citrus fruits such as:

- Lemon
- Lime
- Grapefruit
- Oranges

Melons are best as single ingredient juices:
- Cantaloupe
- Honeydew melon
- Watermelon

Choose a fruit or vegetable with high water content such as:
- Apple
- Beets
- Celery
- Carrot
- Cucumber
- Grapes
- Kiwi
- Pear
- Pineapple

May combine with 1-2 green leafy vegetables such as:
- Collard greens
- Dandelion greens
- Kale
- Mustard greens
- Spinach
- Swiss chard
- Watercress

Add herbs for detoxification / flavor:
- Basil
- Cilantro
- Ginger
- Mint
- Parsley
- Turmeric

Juice is made using a high-powered blender. The whole fruit or vegetable is blended into a liquid.

Pick one base:
- Purified water
- Coconut water
- Herbal tea
- Natural (unpasteurized) fruit juice
- Plant based milk (almond, coconut, etc.)

Add 1-2 vegetables:
- Leafy greens such as kale, romaine lettuce, spinach, watercress, etc.
- 1-2 Tbsp. Irish moss gel
- 1 Tsp powdered vegetables such as beets, chlorella, kelp, irish moss, spirulina, wheatgrass, etc.

Pick one or two fruits to sweeten:
- Berries
- Banana
- Pineapple
- Mango
- Cherries
- Dried fruit (apricots, dates, goji berries etc.)

Add for flavor and/or detoxification (optional):
- Lemon juice
- Handful of fresh herbs (parsley, cilantro, basil, etc)
- Ginger
- Natural sweetener (agave, honey, maple syrup, unsulfured molasses)
- Spices (cinnamon, nutmeg, vanilla)

Add for a boost of energy (optional):
- Raw cacao
- Raw maca powder
- Bee pollen

Add seeds / nuts for more protein or fat (optional):
- Chia seeds
- Hemp seeds
- Flax seeds
- Raw cashews
- Raw almonds
- Raw pumpkin seeds

Tip: Juice should be consumed immediately within 30 minutes of juicing.

Delicious Juice Blends

- Grapefruit, orange, lime citrus juice blend (mucous buster)

- Cucumber, celery, apple juice (kidney flush)

- Carrot, apple, ginger, beet juice (improve circulation)

- Apple, Carrot, Celery, Dandelion Greens, Ginger, Parsley Juice (detoxify)

- Celery, Cucumber, Apple Juice (improve digestion)

- Dandelion Greens, Beetroot, Lemon, Cucumber and Fennel Bulbs Juice (lower cholesterol)

- Kale, Apple, Lemon Juice (alkalinize pH)

- Spinach, Cucumber, Lemon Juice (remineralize bones)

- Swiss Chard, Radish, Ginger, Beet and Kale juice (cancer-fighting)

Infused Water

Directions: Add a combination of favorite fruit and herbs to spring water and soak in mason jar overnight.

- Orange, lime, cucumber, mint

- Strawberry, lemon, basil

- Blueberry, lavender

Natural Fruit Soda

Ingredients:

- 1 cup strawberries (or fruit of your choice), washed and trimmed

- 1 cup carbonated water

- cheesecloth or mesh strainer

Directions: Add strawberries to a food processor and puree until smooth, scraping down the sides of the machine as needed. Use the cheesecloth to strain as much juice as possible, leaving behind the seeds and pulp. Add strawberry puree to the carbonated water. Mix well and serve immediately. To adjust flavor, add lemon juice if too sweet or honey if too tart.

Try these other fruit flavors: mango, pineapple, kiwi, orange, grapefruit, blueberry, peach, or grape.

Jamaican Sea Moss Drink

Ingredients:

- 2 oz Sea Moss
- 1 cup spring water
- 1/4 Tbsp cinnamon
- 1/4 tsp ground nutmeg
- 1/2 tsp vanilla

- 2 cups almond milk
- 1 cup ice
- agave or raw cane sugar to taste
- coconut condensed milk to taste

Directions: Soak for 6-12 hours. Sea Moss will expand to twice its size. After soaking, rinse again and cut into small pieces. Add Sea Moss to a blender with 1 cup spring water and blend to gel consistency. Add water as needed for desired consistency. Pour into a mason jar and set aside. Sea Moss gel may be stored in the refrigerator for several weeks.

Add to blender 1 cup ice, 1 cup almond milk, 3-4 Tbsp Sea Moss gel, cinnamon, and ground nutmeg. Blend to desired thickness and add more almond milk slowly as needed. Add coconut condensed milk and sweetener of choice to taste, and blend well.   Drink immediately.

Piña Colada

Ingredients:

- 1/2 cup coconut milk, full fat
- Juice of 1 lime
- 3 cups frozen pineapple (or 3 cups fresh pineapple with 1 cup ice)
- 4 springs fresh cilantro
- 1-2 cups coconut water, as needed
- 2-3 Tbsp agave syrup or raw cane sugar, sweeten to taste

Directions: Add frozen pineapple, 1 cup coconut water, cilantro, and lime juice to the blender. Blend 2-3 minutes to desired consistency, adding coconut water as needed. Add agave to the mixture to sweeten and blend. Pour into a glass pitcher, serve and enjoy.

TIP: Live food is uncooked, sun-fired, or heated up to 100 degrees in a dehydrator or on the lowest setting in the oven. Food should be served warm from a minimum room temperature (72 degrees) and a maximum of 100º F to maintain live nutrients. Avoid or minimize eating cold foods, which can cause stomach cramping or aggravate painful menstrual cramps in women.

Grand Rising Chia Porridge:

Ingredients:

- 1 cup coconut milk (full fat)
- 1 cup water
- 1/2 tsp vanilla extract
- 3 Tbsp maple syrup
- 1/4 tsp cinnamon powder
- 1/4 tsp ground nutmeg

Directions: In a mixing bowl, combine coconut milk, water, vanilla extract, maple syrup, cinnamon and nutmeg. Whisk in 2 cups chia seeds. Pour mixture into glass container, refrigerate 4-8 hours to let gel. Warm jar in hot water and serve warm.

Strawberries and Cream Smoothie Bowl

Ingredients:

- 1 cup strawberries
- 1/2 cup blueberries
- 1 cup coconut yogurt
- 1 Tbsp maple syrup
- 1/2 tsp vanilla
- 2 Tbsp granola
- 1 Tbsp coconut flakes
- 1 tsp chia seeds
- 1 Tbsp pumpkin seeds

Directions: In Blender, blend 1/2 cup strawberries, coconut yogurt, maple syrup and vanilla. Pour into bowl and top with granola, the rest of strawberries, blueberries, coconut flakes, chia seeds and pumpkin seeds.

Banana Ice Cream

Ingredients:

- 2 ripe bananas, chopped and frozen.

Directions: Blend in food processor or blender. Occasionally scrape down the side and continue blending until smooth. Scoop into a bowl. Add favorite toppings and fruit. Serve immediately.

Honey Nut Oats

Ingredients:

- 1 cup rolled oats
- 1/4 tsp cinnamon
- 1/4 tsp nutmeg
- 1 tsp vanilla
- 1 Tbsp honey (substitute with maple syrup or agave)
- 1 Tbsp. dried cranberries
- ½ Tbsp. raisins
- 1 Tbsp. walnuts

Directions: Fill glass jar halfway with rolled oats. Mix in cinnamon, ground nutmeg, vanilla, raw honey or favorite sweetener. Pour over favorite plant-based milk until oats are covered. Top with raisins, dried cranberries, and walnuts. Soak 30 minutes to 1 hour. Optional: Warm jar in hot water and serve warm.

Coconut Sweet Plantains

Ingredients:

- 2-3 ripe (mostly black skin) sweet plantains
- 1 Tbsp coconut condensed milk
- 1/2 tsp vanilla

Directions: Cut length-wise along the plantains and remove skin. Chop plantain diagonally into 1-inch pieces and set on plate. Drizzle vanilla and coconut condensed milk over plantains to taste, serve and enjoy.

Caribbean Fruit Platter

- Ingredients:
- 3-4 burro bananas, sliced
- 1 medium pineapple, sliced
- 2-3 mangos, sliced
- 1/2 papaya, sliced
- 1 cup rambutan or guineps
- 1-2 cups swan grapes (or other seeded grapes)
- 1-2 pomegranates, sliced into quarters

Directions: Serve on a large decorative platter and enjoy. Serves 2-4.

Banana Berry Cereal

Ingredients:

- 1-2 bananas, chopped

- 1/2- 1 cup mixed berries

- 1-2 Tbsp cacao nibs

- Handful of sprouted buckwheat

- Homemade cashew or almond milk

Directions: Fill a bowl with bananas, berries, cacao nibs, sprouted buckwheat and pour over cashew or almond milk.

Yogurt Parfait

- 2 cups coconut yogurt (or any plant-based yogurt)

- ½ cup granola Granola

- 1 cup berries of choice

- ½ cup shredded coconut

Directions: Fill mason jar halfway with coconut yogurt. Layer with granola, berries and shredded coconut. Enjoy.

Tahini sauce

Ingredients:

- 1/2 cup organic tahini paste

- 1/4 tsp sea salt, plus more to taste

- 1/4 tsp garlic powder

- 1/4 tsp ground black pepper

- 2 Tbsp fresh parsley, minced

- 2 Tbsp fresh lemon juice

- 1/4 cup warm purified water

Directions: Add tahini, sea salt, garlic powder and parsley to mixing bowl and whisk together. Continue to whisk while adding lemon juice. Next, whisk in water until the sauce is a creamy, pourable consistency. Add more salt, pepper, garlic powder or lemon juice to adjust taste to your liking. This sauce adds a mild, creamy flavor to falafels, salads, veggie burgers and live dishes. Store in mason jar and refrigerate for 1-2 weeks.

Carrot "Tuna"

Inspired by Queen Afua

Ingredients:

- 7 medium-sized carrots
- 1/4 cup vegan mayonnaise
- 1-2 scallions, diced
- 1 stalk celery, diced
- 1/2 one red pepper, diced

- 3 sprigs fresh parsley, diced
- 1 tsp kelp granules
- 1/2 tsp garlic powder
- 1/2 tsp celery salt
- 1/2 tsp ground black pepper

Directions: Juice the carrots. Pour the juice in a mason jar and refrigerate. Place the pulp aside in a large mixing bowl for the carrot tuna salad. Add all other ingredients to the carrot pulp and mix well. Serve over seaweed wrap, lettuce or sprouted toast.

Simple Moroccan Couscous

Ingredients:

- 1 cup couscous, uncooked
- 1 cup vegetable broth, warm
- 1 tsp ground cumin
- 2 Tbsp lemon juice

- 1/4 tsp sea salt
- 1/4 tsp ground black pepper
- Few sprigs of fresh parsley and basil (or herb of choice), finely chopped
- 1 Tbsp olive oil

Directions: In a small mixing bowl add dried couscous, cumin, sea salt, pepper, parsley and basil. Combine ingredients well. Add lemon juice and mix well.   Drizzle over oil and mix well. Pour over vegetable broth, cover and let sit for 30 minutes until couscous expands to twice its size. Plate and serve.

Creamy Kale Salad

Ingredients:

- 1/4 head cabbage, thinly sliced
- 3 carrots, peeled and shredded
- 1 granny smith apple, shredded
- 1/2 pound kale, finely chopped
- 1 recipe cashew herb dressing (recipe below)

Directions: Prepare cashew herb dressing and set aside. Add cabbage, carrots, apple and kale to a large bowl and set aside. Pour over cashew herb dressing. Mix well, serve and enjoy.

Cashew Herb Dressing

Ingredients:

- 1 cup cashews, soaked in water for 4-8 hours
- 1/4 cup raw hulled hemp seeds
- 1/4 cup fresh dill, chopped
- 1/4 cup fresh chives, chopped
- 1/4 cup parsley, chopped
- 1/4 cup nutritional yeast
- 3 cloves garlic, chopped
- Juice of 1/2 lemon
- Salt and pepper to taste
- water as needed

Directions: In a blender, add 1/2 cup water, cashews and remaining ingredients. Blend to desired smooth consistency, adding more water as needed.

Seaweed Salad

Ingredients:

- Nori seaweed, 20 sheets
- 3 Tbsp liquid aminos
- 3 Tbsp sesame seeds, roasted
- 3 Tbsp sesame oil
- 3 Tbsp water

Directions: In a large mixing bowl, take 1-2 sheets of nori at a time, and rip into small 1-2" pieces. Add liquid aminos and water, and use hands to massage into the nori, moistening all the pieces. Add sesame seeds and sesame oil to mixture, and continue massaging in to combine ingredients well. Serve as a side with dish of your choice.

Vegan Alfredo Sauce

Ingredients:

- 1 cup cashews soaked overnight for 6 hours (substitute with walnuts or pine nuts)

- 3 Tbsp Nutritional yeast

- 2 cloves garlic, minced

- 2 Tbsp onions, diced

- 1 pinch sea salt and black pepper

- 1 handful fresh basil

- 1 cup purified water

Note: For a cooked vegetarian option and quicker preparation, bring cashews to a boil, then let simmer and cook for 20 minutes until soft.

Directions: Add dry ingredients into a high powered blender with 1 cup water. Blend ingredients well, adding more lemon juice as needed until desired creamy consistency is achieved.

Garlic Alfredo Zucchini Pasta

Ingredients:

- 4-5 zucchinis

- 1 pinch black pepper

- 1 tsp fresh basil, chopped

- 1 recipe for vegan Alfredo sauce

Directions: Spiralize zucchinis for noodles and set aside. Prepare 1 recipe of vegan Alfredo sauce and pour over noodles. Sprinkle over black pepper to taste, garnish with fresh basil, serve and enjoy.

Creole Cauliflower Wings

Ingredients:

- 1-2 large heads of cauliflower cut into the size of wings

- 2 cups cherry tomatoes

- 4-5 carrots, chopped

- 1 tsp chili pepper

- 1 Tbsp cumin

- 1 Tbsp paprika

- 1 Tbsp cayenne pepper

- 1 thumb ginger

- 1 lemon, juiced

- few springs of cilantro

Directions: Place cauliflower in a large bowl and set aside. In high powered blender, blend to desired consistency 2 cups cherry tomatoes, 4-5 carrots, 1 Tbsp. cumin, 1 Tbsp paprika, 1 Tbsp cayenne pepper, 1 thumb ginger, lemon juice, cilantro. Mix well until cauliflower is completely covered. Place in dehydrator for 8 hours until dry or in oven on lowest temperature for 2-3 hours.

No-Bake Stuffed Peppers

Ingredients:

- 4 bell or poblano peppers, cut in half

- 1 cup raw cashews, soaked 4-6 hours

- 1 cup raw sunflower seeds

- 2 sprigs fresh dill, chopped

- 2 sprigs fresh cilantro, chopped

- 1 lemon, juiced

Directions: Blend raw cashews, sunflower seeds, dill, cilantro, and lemon juice to creamy consistency. Fill peppers with cashew blend. Top with chopped herbs and serve.

Collard Greens

Ingredients:

- 1 bunch collard greens, washed
- 2 Tbsp olive oil
- 1/4 cup apple cider vinegar
- 6-8 sun-dried tomatoes, chopped
- 1/2 onion, chopped
- 2 cloves garlic, minced
- 1tsp paprika
- 1/2 tsp black pepper
- 1/2 tsp cayenne pepper
- 1/2 tsp salt

Directions: Remove the leaves of the collard greens from the stems. Stack 3-4 leaves onto each other and roll length-wise into cylinder shape. Cut along the collards 1" apart, making strips. Add collard strips to a large bowl. Pour over olive oil and sprinkle on salt. Use hands to mix well and massage mixture into greens. Add sun-dried tomatoes, garlic, onions, then sprinkle over paprika, black pepper, and cayenne pepper. Combine ingredients well. Pout over apple cider vinegar. Mix well and massage into collard greens. Let marinate in refrigerator for 4 hours or overnight.

Veggie Pizza

Crust:

- 1 cup raw cauliflower
- 2 medium zucchinis
- 1 cup mushrooms
- 2 scallions
- 1 cup fresh basil
- 1 cup fresh cooking sage
- 1 Tbsp. thyme
- 1 handful spinach

Marinara sauce:

- 2 heirloom tomatoes, chopped
- ½ cup sun-dried tomatoes
- ½ cup red bell pepper, chopped
- ½ cup firmly packed basil leaves
- 2 Tbsp. cold-pressed olive oil
- 1 Tbsp. fresh lemon juice
- 1 Tbsp red onion, finely chopped
- 1 clove fresh garlic, minced

Vegan Cheese:

- 1 yellow zucchini, shredded

- 3 Tbsp nutritional yeast

- 1 Tbsp fresh lemon juice

- 1 tsp garlic powder

- A pinch salt

Directions: Blend together all ingredients for crust until smooth. Pour onto parchment paper in 6" circle and place in dehydrator for 10-12 hours at 100°F or in the oven on the lowest temperature for 6-8 hours. For marinara sauce, combine together in a food processor cherry tomatoes, sun-dried tomatoes, red bell pepper, basil, olive oil, lemon juice, red onion, minced garlic in food processor or blender to desired consistency. Pour sauce over pizza crust and spread evenly. Combine ingredients for vegan cheese and sprinkle on top of marinara sauce. Top with fresh herbs of choice, slice evenly into 8 pieces and enjoy.

Tabouli

Ingredients:

- 1 cup bulgar wheat

- 2 heirloom tomatoes

- 1 cucumber

- 2 bunches parsley washed & dried

- 12-15 mint leaves

- 4 scallions

- 1/4 tsp sea salt

- 3-4 Tbsp lime juice

- 3-4 Tbsp olive oil

Directions: Soak 1 cup bulgar wheat for 30 min. Drain well to remove excess water. Finely chop 4 firm roma tomatoes, 1 cucumber, 2 bunches parsley washed & dried, 12-15 mint leaves, 4 scallions, 1/4 tsp sea salt 3-4 Tbsp lime juice, 3-4 Tbsp olive oil. Mix ingredients well, refrigerate 30 min and serve.

Live "Sautéed" Mushrooms

Ingredients:

- 2 cups Shiitake mushrooms (or any mushroom of choice), cut into 1" slices
- 1 Tbsp Spike Natural seasoning, to taste
- 1 tsp Fresh or dried parsley
- 1 Tbsp Balsamic Vinegar
- 2 Tbsp Olive oil

Directions: In a large mixing bowl, add mushrooms, parsley and spike seasoning and combine. Pour over balsamic vinegar, and olive oil. Mix ingredients well. Marinate in refrigerator for 4 hours and serve.

Carrot Apple Beet Salad

Ingredients:

- 1 large carrot, peeled and tops removed
- 1 apple, peeled and core removed
- 1 beet, peeled

Dressing:

- 2 cloves garlic, chopped
- 2 Tbsp olive oil
- Sea salt and pepper to taste
- 1 thumb ginger, chopped
- 1 Tbsp honey
- Juice of 1 orange
- Juice and zest of 2 lemons

Directions: Shred carrots, apples and beets using a grater or food processor. To make the dressing add orange, and lemon juices, garlic, honey, and olive oil to a blender. Sprinkle in a pinch of salt and pepper. Blend well. Pour desired amount of dressing over salad, combine ingredients and serve.

Hot Pepper Gazpacho

Ingredients:

- 3-4 large heirloom tomatoes, chopped
- ½ -1 tsp. red pepper flakes
- 1-2 tsp. garlic powder
- ½ tsp. Himalayan salt
- 1 tsp. ground Annatto
- 1 tsp. ground black pepper
- Onion, diced
- Dill, chopped
- 1 red pepper, chopped
- 1 sprig cilantro, chopped

Directions: Add to blender tomatoes, onions, red pepper, dill and cilantro, and blend on low speed. Increase speed slowly to blend ingredients to thick, chunky consistency. Add red pepper flakes, garlic powder, Himalayan salt, annatto, black pepper and continue blending, adjusting speed to blend soup to desired consistency. Bowl and serve.

Guacamole

Ingredients:

- 3 avocados
- 1 lime, juiced
- 1 tsp. sea salt
- 1 clove garlic, minced
- ½ cup onion, diced
- ¼ tsp. (or less) ground cayenne pepper
- 1 sprig cilantro, finely chopped
- 2 roma tomatoes, diced

Directions: In a medium bowl, add the avocado, lime juice and salt. Mash together well. Add in garlic, onion, cayenne pepper, tomatoes, and cilantro. Mix and combine well. Serve as a dip or on your favorite wrap or sandwich.

Cucumber Tacos

Ingredients:

- 2 cucumbers, sliced in half length-wise, insides scooped out
- 1 large heirloom tomato, chopped
- 1 sprig fresh dill, finely chopped
- 1 shallot, chopped
- ½ avocado, chopped
- 1 tsp. finely chopped jalapeño pepper
- 1 ½ lemon
- 1 tsp. spike seasoning
- 1 tsp. paprika
- 1 tsp. ground red pepper
- ½ tsp. nutritional yeast (optional)

Directions: In a large mixing bowl, add tomato, dill, shallots, avocado and jalapeño pepper and combine well. Add spike seasoning, paprika, ground red pepper and squeeze lemon juice over the mixture. Mix well. Scoop out mixture with a spoon and fill cucumbers. Sprinkle over nutritional yeast and serve.

Live Vegan Lasagna

Cheese sauce:

- 1 cup raw macadamia nuts

- 2 Tbsp lime juice

- 3/4 cup almond milk

- pinch salt and pepper

- 2 Tbsp nutritional yeast flakes

- 2 sprigs thyme

Directions: Soak the macadamia nuts for 4-6 hours. Drain the water from the macadamia nuts and transfer the nuts to the blender. Add the almond milk, lemon juice, nutritional yeast, thyme, salt and pepper and blend to a creamy, smooth sauce. Set aside in refrigerator.

Tomato sauce:

- 1 large heirloom tomato, chopped

- 1/4 cup water

- 1 Tbsp fresh lemon juice

- 1 Tbsp basil, chopped

- 1/2 garlic clove

- 1 tsp oregano

- 1 Tbsp agave syrup

- 1 Tbsp sun-dried tomato, chopped

Directions: Add to a blender the fresh tomato, sun-dried tomatoes, agave syrup, lemon juice, basil, garlic, and oregano. Combine well by pulsing mixture to a chunky texture, adding water slowly. Pulse to desired consistency. Set aside.

Pesto Sauce:

- 1/2 cup pine nuts (substitute with walnuts)
- handful fresh basil
- handful fresh parsley
- 1/2 avocado
- 2 Tbsp extra-virgin olive oil
- 1/2 cup water
- 2 Tbsp fresh lemon juice
- pinch sea salt and pepper

Directions: Add pine nuts, basil, parsley, avocado, olive oil, lemon juice, salt and pepper, to blender with 1/4 cup water. Blend until smooth consistency, adding water slowly as needed. Set aside.

Vegetable layers:

- 2 zucchinis, sliced into long thin strips as lasagna noodles
- 2 large heirloom tomatoes, cut into thin slices
- handful of basil
- handful of spinach

Directions: In a 9 x 13" lasagna pan, first create the bottom layer with the zucchini noodles. Moving upward, layer the tomatoes, spinach, tomato sauce, cheese sauce and pesto. Repeat with another layer starting with the zucchini noodles and finishing with the pesto sauce. Top with basil leaves and pine nuts to garnish. Serve fresh.

Jamaican Sorrel Drink

- 8 oz dried sorrel

- 6 cups purified water

- 2 thumbs ginger, chopped

- 1 tsp cloves

- 1 tsp allspice

- 3-4 sticks cinnamon

- 1/2 tsp nutmeg

- 1 cup raw cane sugar (or agave syrup) to taste

Directions: Add sorrel, purified water, ginger, cloves, cinnamon and nutmeg into large pot and bring to a boil. Let simmer over medium heat for 30 minutes. Turn off flame and let cool. Strain sorrel and add raw cane sugar to taste. Mix well until sugar is dissolved. Refrigerate and serve cool or over ice.

Pineapple Ginger Drink

Inspired by Elsie Obed

Ingredients:

- 1 large ripe pineapple, peeled and diced

- 2 thumbs fresh peeled ginger, diced

- 1 tsp cloves

- 1 cup raw cane sugar (or agave syrup) to taste

- Juice of 1 medium-sized lime or 2 Tbsp lime juice

- 6 cups spring water

Directions: Blend pineapple and ginger with 1 cup water until smooth and pour in a large pot. Add cloves and pour in 6 cups spring water. Bring to a boil, then simmer over medium heat for 30 minutes. Turn off flame and let cool. Strain mixture using cheesecloth or fine sieve and add lime juice.   Add sugar and mix well until sugar is dissolved. Refrigerate, serve over ice and enjoy!

Green Banana Porridge

Ingredients:

- 3 green bananas
- 2 1/2 cups water
- 2 cups almond milk
- 2 Tbsp coconut condensed milk
- 1 tsp vanilla extract
- 1/4 tsp nutmeg
- 1/4 tsp cinnamon
- 1/8 tsp sea salt
- *optional- add natural cane sugar to taste

Directions: Wash green bananas. Cut the tips off, make an incision length-wise and remove the peel. Grate the banana using the large side of the grater. Add the grated bananas into a large saucepan, bring to a boil and reduce heat while stirring. Stir in coconut milk and spices and let cook over medium heat until ingredients are blended well. Stir occasionally until consistency is smooth. Let simmer for 5 minute and serve warm.

Blueberry Waffles

Ingredients:

- 2 cups whole wheat flour
- 1 Tbsp baking powder
- 1/4 tsp Himalayan pink salt or sea salt
- Vegan egg-replacer equivalent to 3 eggs
- 1/4 tsp cinnamon
- A pinch of nutmeg
- 1 tsp vanilla
- 1 1/2 cup almond milk
- 1 Tbsp grapeseed oil
- 1/2 cup blueberries

Directions: Sift the flour into a large mixing bowl. Add the baking powder, salt, vegan egg replacer, cinnamon and nutmeg. Mix dry ingredients well. Add almond milk, vanilla and grapeseed oil. Combine well together with dry ingredients until batter is smooth and creamy without lumps. Pour batter into waffle maker, place blueberries in each waffle, and follow the manufacturer's instructions.

Nutty Quinoa Cereal

Ingredients:

- 2 cups almond milk (or any plant-based milk)
- 1 cup quinoa, rinsed
- 3 Tbsp agave (or desired natural sweetener)
- 1/4 tsp cinnamon
- 1/4 tsp ground nutmeg
- A dash of vanilla extract
- 3 Tbsp dried fruit (raisins, cherries, cranberries)
- 2 Tbsp toasted pecans

Directions: Bring quinoa and almond milk to a boil in a medium saucepan. Reduce to low heat and simmer, covered for 15 minutes. Add agave, cinnamon, nutmeg, vanilla extract and dried fruit. Mix well and continue to simmer, uncovered, until most of the almond milk has been absorbed (about 5-7 minutes). Remove from heat, spoon into bowls and top with toasted pecans.

Ackee No Salt-fish (a vegan ackee recipe)

1 lb ackee (use frozen ackee if fresh ackee is unavailable in your country or canned ackee in brine if neither fresh nor frozen ackee is available)

- 1 1/2 cups mushrooms (diced)
- 1/4 onion diced
- 1/2 cup red peppers
- 1 garlic clove (minced)
- 2 tsp dried parsley
- 1/2 tsp smoked paprika
- 1/2 tsp dry mustard
- 1/2 tsp turmeric
- 1/4 tsp cumin
- 1/2 tsp Himalayan pink salt
- 1/8 tsp pepper
- 1 tsp nutritional yeast
- 1 Tbsp grapeseed oil

Directions: Fresh ackee: Add to a medium saucepan with 1 cup spring water with a pinch of salt. Bring to a boil and cook for 15 minutes until tender. Drain water and set ackee aside.

Frozen ackee: Let thaw or bring to a boil in spring water for 10 minutes until tender, drain and set aside

Canned ackee: Drain salt water. Rinse, drain and set aside.

Heat grapeseed oil in a skillet over medium heat. Add onion, red peppers and garlic to skillet and sauté for 2 minutes. Add the mushrooms and sauté 1-2 minutes. Add ackee and combine well. Sprinkle over dried parsley, dry mustard, turmeric, cumin, paprika sea salt, pepper. Mix well and sauté for 3-4 minutes and let the flavors meld. Serve hot.

Note: Fresh ackee is banned from importing to the U.S. To prepare fresh ackee, ensure the fruit is fully mature and naturally ripened. Fully mature ackee is yellow and red color with no green and opens naturally, exposing the seeds and arils. The inside of the pod becomes visible, and the pod begins to shrivel. Only at this time is ackee suitable for eating. Ackee that is not fully mature and opened naturally on its own is inedible and poisonous. To clean the fully mature ackee: remove the pieces from the seed pod, then separate the seed, membrane and aril. Keep the arils and discard the rest. Rinse, drain and prepare as directed above.

Green Bananas

Ingredients:

6 to 8 green bananas

water

salt

Directions: Wash the green bananas. Use a paring knife to cut off both ends of each banana. Make two cuts lengthwise along each banana. Fill a large pot two-thirds full of water. Add a dash of salt. Bring the water to a boil over medium-high heat. Place the whole, unpeeled green bananas in the boiling water. Allow them to boil for 20 minutes or until soft enough to be easily pierced with a fork. Drain and serve warm.

Jamaican Steamed Cabbage

Ingredients:

1 head of white cabbage

1 medium onion, chopped

1 medium carrot, chopped into thin strips

1 tomato, chopped

2 cloves garlic, minced

1/2 red sweet bell pepper, chopped

1/2 yellow sweet bell pepper

2 springs of thyme

2 Tbsp grapeseed oil

1/4 tsp black pepper

sea salt to taste

1/2 scotch bonnet pepper (optional)

Directions: Cut the cabbage into four quarters, remove the middle, wash the cabbage leaves, slice into small pieces. Set aside. Add grapeseed oil, onion, garlic, scotch bonnet pepper (whole), and thyme to a medium saucepan on medium heat and let cook until onion is soft. Add the tomato and bell pepper. Sauté for 1-2 minutes. Add the cabbage with black pepper and salt. Stir well. Turn heat to low, cover saucepan, and let vegetables cook down half-way done for about 10 minutes. Add the carrots and let vegetables steam until soft and tender or to desired crispness for about 5-10 more minutes. Turn off heat and serve warm.

Sautéed Spinach

Ingredients:

- 16 oz chopped spinach
- 1 plum tomato chopped
- 1/2 medium onion, sliced
- 2 cloves garlic, finely chopped
- 6 medium chestnut mushrooms, chopped
- 3 sprigs fresh thyme

- 1/4 Scotch bonnet pepper
- 1/4 tsp black
- 1/4 tsp spike seasoning (or all-purpose seasoning of choice)
- grapeseed oil

Directions: In a sauté pan add a drizzle of grapeseed oil with onion and garlic over low heat. Add thyme and scotch bonnet pepper. Stir for 3 minutes. Stir in tomato, bell pepper and mushrooms. Cover to simmer for 5 minutes under tender. Add and stir in spinach and spike seasoning. Simmer until spinach is cooked. Serve with steamed cabbage, green bananas and avocado. Enjoy!

Oatmeal Casserole

Ingredients:

- 3 cups stone cut oats
- 1 tsp sea sea
- 1/2 cup coconut
- 1/4 cup sunflower seeds
- 4 cups hot coconut milk
- 1/4 cup almond meal
- 1/2 cup raisins
- 3 Tbsp. honey or agave (optional)

Directions: Combine ingredients and stir. Pour in a casserole dish. Bake at 370°F for 35 minutes until the top is slightly brown.

Vegan Banana Nut Bread

Ingredients:

- 1 cup cane sugar
- 3 medium ripe bananas, mashed
- 1/2 cup unrefined coconut oil, melted
- 1 tsp vanilla
- 1/4 cup unsweetened vanilla almond milk (or plant-based milk)
- 2 cups all-purpose whole grain flour
- 3/4 tsp baking powder
- 1/2 tsp salt
- 1/2 cup chopped walnuts

Directions: Heat oven to 350°F. Grease 9x5x3 inch loaf baking pan. In a large mixing bowl, combine sugar, bananas, coconut oil and vanilla until smooth. Stir in almond milk and use a hand mixer to combine ingredients well. Slowly add flour, baking powder and salt and continue mixing until smooth with no lumps. Fold in walnuts stir well with wooden spoon. Pour into pan. Bake 1 hour or until inserted toothpick comes out clean. Allow to cool, loosen sides from loaf pan, slice and serve.

Hot breakfast Couscous

Ingredients:

- 1 cup coconut milk and 1 cup water (or 2 cups plant-based milk of choice)
- 2 Tbsp agave syrup
- 1 tsp ground cinnamon
- 1 tsp ground nutmeg
- 1/2 tsp vanilla
- 2 cups dry couscous
- 1/3 cup chopped dried apricots
- 1/3 cup raisins
- 1/2 cup slivered almonds

Directions: In a saucepan over medium heat, combine the coconut milk, water. Bring to a boil, stir in couscous. Simmer over medium heat, and stir in apricots and raisins. Add and mix in nutmeg, cinnamon, and agave. Add almonds and mix well. Turn off heat, cover and let stand for 5 minutes. Serve and enjoy!

Live option: Combine couscous with 1/2 cup water, 1/2 cup coconut milk, apricots, raisins, agave, cinnamon and vanilla in bowl or large mason jar. Soak for 15-20 minutes until couscous expands to twice its volume. Warm 1/2 cup water with 1/2 cup coconut milk. Pour over couscous mixture, and mix well. Top with almonds. Serve and enjoy!

Simple Vegetable Broth

Ingredients:

- 2 stalks celery, chopped
- 5 springs fresh thyme
- 2 onions, chopped
- 1 sprig scallion, chopped
- 1 fennel bulb, chopped
- 8 cloves garlic minced
- 3 bay leaves
- 1 tsp salt
- 2 quarts purified water
- 1 tsp whole black peppercorns
- 1 Tbsp grapeseed oil
- 4 quarts purified water

Directions: Heat the grapeseed oil in a large stockpot over medium heat. Add vegetables and spices and let cook, stirring occasionally until vegetables begin to soften. Add 4 quarts water and bring to a boil. Reduce heat and let simmer until broth is reduced by half, 60 to 90 minutes. Strain broth through a fine sieve. Store in the fridge 3-4 days or up to 6 months in the freezer.

Jamaican Dumplings

Ingredients:

- 1/2 cup all-purpose whole grain wheat flour
- 1/4 cup water
- pinch sea salt

Note: This recipe can be prepared as boiled dumplings or as fried dumpling festival.

Directions: Place flour and salt in mixing bowl. Add water and mix to make a stiff dough. Pinch off small pieces of dough. For round dumplings, roll dough into a ball in the palm of hand then gently press your thumb into the middle of the ball to slightly flatten into 2" round dumpling. For long dumplings, roll dough in the palm of hands to make 1" thick and 2" long.

To cook: add dumplings to cook in stew, boil in water with a pinch of sea salt to serve as side dish or fry in coconut oil to make Jamaican fried dumpling festival.

Ital Stew Peas

Ingredients:

- 2 cups dried kidney beans
- 6 cups water
- 2 cups coconut milk
- 1 onion, minced and/or 2 scallions chopped
- 2 cloves garlic, minced
- 1 carrot, diced

- 1 spring thyme
- 1 whole scotch bonnet pepper with stem intact
- 1/4 tsp fresh ginger grated (optional)
- 1/4 tsp ground allspice
- 1 recipe for dumplings

Directions: Rinse beans and soak overnight for 8 hours. Discard water and rinse beans with fresh water. Place in large saucepan with water and bring to boil. Lower heat to simmer until tender for 1 hour. Add coconut milk, carrots, onion, garlic and continue simmering. Add dumplings, thyme and other spices. Simmer for 30 minutes until sauce is thick. Discard pepper before serving. Serve with brown rice and mixed greens salad.

Spicy Black Bean Veggie Burgers

Burger:

- 1 1/2 cup black beans, cooked
- 1/4 cup finely chopped cilantro
- 1 tsp ground cumin
- 1 tsp ground coriander
- 1/4 tsp cayenne pepper
- 1 clove garlic

- 1 cup cooked quinoa, cooled
- sea salt
- freshly ground black pepper to taste
- 2 Tbsp chia seeds (vegan egg replacer)
- 1 Tbsp grapeseed oil

Spicy Mayonaise Sauce:

- 1/2 cup vegan mayonnaise
- 1 1/2 tsp Old Bay seasoning
- 1 tsp lemon juice
- 1/2 tsp hot sauce

For serving:

- 4 whole-wheat hamburger buns, toasted
- Avocado slices
- 1 cup caramelized onions
- romaine lettuce

Directions: Preheat oven to 375°F. Place Chia seeds in bowl, add 1 cup hot water, set aside. In a food processor, combine beans, cilantro, cumin, coriander, cayenne, and garlic. Pulse until slightly chunky. Transfer mixture into a large bowl, add quinoa. Season with salt and pepper. Mix in chia seeds and combine. Divide mixture into 4 balls. Place on a large plate and gently flatten to form patties. Cover with plastic wrap and transfer to the fridge to set for 10 minutes. In a small bowl whisk together vegan mayonnaise, Old bay seasoning, lemon juice and hot sauce. Season to taste with salt and pepper. Drizzle grapeseed oil in large sauté pan and sear burgers for 2-3 minutes each side over medium heat. Then place in oven for 10 to 12 minutes until cooked through. Serve burgers on hamburger buns with a tsp. of spicy mayonnaise sauce, topped with caramelized onions, avocado, and romaine lettuce.

Stuffed Portobello Mushrooms

Ingredients:

- 4 large portobello mushrooms caps
- 4 Tbsps grape seed oil
- 1 clove garlic peeled and minced
- 1 small onion, caramelized
- 1 green or red bell pepper finely diced
- 3-4 leaves of kale, stems removed, finely chopped

- 1 cup cooked quinoa
- 2 sprigs dill finely chopped
- 2 Tbsp nutritional yeast
- 1/2 tsp paprika
- 1/2 tsp ground black pepper
- 1 pinch Himalayan sea salt

Directions: Preheat oven to 400 degrees F. Line a baking sheet with parchment paper and place the mushroom caps facing up. Brush each with grape seed oil and set aside. In a large pan over medium-high heat, add remaining grapeseed oil, garlic and peppers and stir fry for 2 minutes.   Add kale and dill and stir fry for 2 minutes until vegetables are tender but still yielding a soft crunch. Sprinkle over paprika, salt and pepper. Fill each mushroom with 1-2 Tbsp each of quinoa, stir-fried vegetables, and caramelized onions. Bake in oven for 8-10 minutes until mushrooms soften. Serve warm and enjoy.

Grilled Jerk Eggplant Steaks

Eggplant:

- 1 tsp ground cinnamon
- 1 Tbsp ground coriander
- 1/4 tsp allspice
- 1/4 tsp cayenne pepper
- 1/2 tsp each sea salt and black pepper
- 2 Tbsp fresh thyme
- 4 cloves garlic, minced
- 1Tbsp fresh grated ginger
- 3 Tbsp lime juice

- 1/4 cup tamari or coconut aminos
- 2-3 Tbsp coconut sugar or maple syrup to taste
- 2 Tbsp melted coconut oil, plus more for grilling
- 3 scallions thinly sliced
- 1 thinly sliced Serrano or habanero pepper, seeds removed
- 1 large or 2 small eggplants

Directions: In a mixing bowl, mix together cinnamon, coriander, allspice, cayenne, salt, pepper, thyme, garlic, ginger, lime juice, tamari, maple syrup, coconut oil, scallions and Serrano pepper. Taste and adjust flavor as needed, adding more tamari for saltiness, line juice for acidity, fresh herbs for earthy flavor, maple syrup for sweetness, pepper for heat or garlic for bite/zing. Slice eggplant lengthwise into 1/2 inch steaks and generously brush both sides with the marinade. Heat up a cast-iron grill medium-high heat and lightly oil. Wrap each eggplant steak in foil and grill for 3-5 minutes on each side until golden brown.

BBQ Jackfruit Sliders

- 5 lb. fresh unripe jackfruit
- 1/2 cup vegan BBQ sauce
- 3 cloves garlic, minced
- 1 tsp sea salt
- 1 tsp ground black pepper
- 1/2 tsp paprika
- 1 tsp liquid smoke
- 1 tsp ground red pepper
- 1 tsp tamari
- 2 tsp molasses or brown sugar
- 1 Tbsp grapeseed oil
- 1 cup vegetable broth

Directions: Preheat oven to 400 degrees. Prepare fresh, unripe jackfruit by removing the skin and outer 1/4 to 1/2 of the jackfruit. Pull apart the stringy parts of the jackfruit, discard the rest and set aside. In a medium saucepan heat the grapeseed oil and add the onions to cook for 3-4 minutes. Add the garlic, salt and pepper for 1-2 minutes until flavors meld. Add the jackfruit, paprika, ground red pepper, liquid smoke, tamarin and brown sugar, and mix well. Add the vegetable broth, cover pot and let simmer over medium heat for 15 minutes until jackfruit is soft and liquid is mostly absorbed.

Remove from flame and transfer to baking sheet lined with parchment paper. Place in oven and bake for 20 minutes. Cover jackfruit in BBQ sauce, mix well and bake for another 10 minutes until lightly brown. Remove jackfruit from oven. Serve on bread rolls, top with coleslaw and serve warm.

Falafel Balls

Ingredients:

- 2 cups chickpeas, cooked, drained and patted dry
- 1/3 cup chopped fresh parsley (or cilantro)
- 4 cloves garlic, minced
- 2 shallots, minced
- 2 Tbsp raw sesame seeds

- 1 1/2 tsp cumin, plus more to taste

- 1/2 tsp each sea salt and pepper, plus more to taste

- A pinch each of cardamom and coriander (optional)

- 3-4 Tbsp all-purpose whole whole flour (or gluten-free alternative)

- 3-4 Tbsp grapeseed oil for cooking

- Panko bread crumbs for coating (optional)

Directions: Add chickpeas, parsley, shallots, garlic, sesame seeds, cumin, salt, pepper, coriander and cardamom to a food processor or blender and mix/pulse to combine into a crumbly dough (not a paste), scraping down sides as needed. Add flour 1 tbsp at a time and pulse/mix to combine until no longer wet and you can mold the dough into a ball without it sticking to your hands.

Transfer to a mixing bowl, cover and refrigerate for 1-2 hours (you may skip this step in if in a hurry). Once chilled, scoop out, mix 1 Tbsp at a time and gently form into small balls. Sprinkle on bread crumbs for crispier crust. Heat a large skillet over medium heat with 1-2 Tbsp grapeseed oil and add falafels. Cook for 4-5 minutes until golden brown, turning occasionally. Serve over whole-grain pasta (may use gluten-free or zucchini noodles) and marinara sauce, or with hummus over a bed of greens.

Baked Cauliflower Chick'n Wings

Cauliflower:

- 1 head of cauliflower, cut into large florets
- 1 cup arrowroot flour
- ½ cup coconut milk (or plant-based milk of choice)
- 1 tsp. garlic powder
- 1 tsp. Old Bay seasoning
- 1 tsp. onion powder
- ½ tsp. chili powder
- ½ tsp. sea salt
- ½ tsp. pepper

Sauce:

- 1/2 cup coconut aminos
- 1/2 freshly squeezed orange juice
- 1/4 cup fire apple cider vinegar and honey tonic
- 2 Tbsp orange zest
- 1/2 tsp ground ginger
- 1/4 tsp crushed red pepper flakes
- 1 Tbsp arrowroot flour

Directions: To make sauce, place all sauce ingredient in a saucepan over medium heat. Let simmer for 15 minutes until sauce thickens, stirring occasionally. Set aside. Preheat oven to 450°F. Line a baking sheet with parchment paper and set aside. Mix together arrowroot flour, garlic powder, chili powder, salt and pepper in a mixing bowl. Slowly whisk in coconut milk until smooth and lump-free. Place cauliflower florets in a large bowl and pour batter on top. Mix thoroughly until coated well. Place florets on baking sheet, shaking off excess batter. Bake for 20 minutes. Take out of oven, let cool for 5 minutes. Place florets in a large bowl and coat each piece thoroughly in sauce. Place back on parchment paper and bake for another 10 minutes. Heat oven to broil, brush remaining sauce on each floret and place in oven for 2-3 minutes. Serve with your choice of greens.

BBQ Mushroom Skewers

Ingredients:

- 2 portobello mushrooms
- 1/2 cup vegan BBQ sauce
- 1/4 cup spring water
- 1 tsp sea salt
- 1 tsp onion powder
- 1/2 tsp cayenne
- grapeseed oil
- basting brush
- skewers (optional)

This recipe can be grilled, cooked in a skillet or baked at 350°F for 10-15 minutes.

Directions: Scrape gills off the underside of each mushroom cap. Slice mushrooms about 1/2 inch apart. Add mushrooms to a large container, add spices, water and BBQ sauce. Cover with a lid, shake and marinate in refrigerator for 6-8 hours. Take a skewer and push through 3 mushrooms around the middle onto each skewer. Place each skewer on lightly oiled cast iron griddle over medium heat. Grill ribs for 12-15 minutes, turning occasionally until lightly brown. Brush as desired with more BBQ sauce. Serve with side dish of choice.

Mac-N- Vegan Cheese

Ingredients:

- 1 cup almond milk
- 2 cups whole grain elbow noodles
- 2 Tbsp vegan butter spread
- 1/2 cup apple sauce
- 2 Tbsp mustard
- 2 Tbsp parsley
- 1 Tbsp paprika
- 1 tsp cayenne pepper
- 1 tsp garlic powder
- 1 tsp sea salt

- 1 tsp black pepper
- 1/4 cup nutritional yeast
- 1 large sweet potato
- 1/2 lb pumpkin
- 2 large carrots, chopped
- 4 quarts purified water

Directions: Preheat oven to 350° F. Add 2 cups purified water to a large saucepan and bring to a boil. Once boiling, add 2 cups pasta and cook pasta halfway. [*Do not fully cook the pasta or the final result will be mushy*]. Drain, rinse in cold water and set aside in a large mixing bowl.

In a separate large saucepan, add 2 quartz purified water with the sweet potato, pumpkin and carrots and bring to a boil. Cook vegetables halfway, strain and add to blender with almond milk. Blend to smooth, creamy consistency. Add mixture to noodles with remaining ingredients and combine well. Pour mixture into baking pan, sprinkle with parsley and paprika. Place in oven and bake for 45 minutes to 1 hour. Let cool for 20 minutes and serve.

Turn Cornmeal

Ingredients:

- 2 cups fine cornmeal
- 2 cups coconut milk
- 2 cups spring water
- 1 cup pumpkin, diced
- 3 cloves garlic minced
- 1 small onion, chopped
- 2 scallions, chopped
- 4 sprigs fresh thyme (or 1 tsp dried)
- 1/4 tsp ground allspice
- 1/2 tsp garlic powder
- 1 Tbsp vegan butter spread
- 1 tsp sea salt
- 1 tsp ground black pepper
- 1 scotch bonnet pepper

Directions: Bring 2 cups water and coconut milk to a boil. Add pumpkin, garlic, onion, scallion, thyme, and scotch bonnet pepper. In a mixing bowl combine cornmeal, garlic powder, sea salt, black pepper and allspice. Once pumpkin is half-way cooked, sift cornmeal mixture into the boiling liquid stirring constantly until the mixture thickens. Cook for 10 minutes until liquid is mostly absorbed. Allow mixture to set and serve.

Oven Roasted Sweet Plantains

Ingredients:

- 2 ripe plantains (very ripe with black spots)

- 2 Tbsp coconut oil

- sea salt to taste

Directions: Cut plantains in half lengthwise, peel and remove the skin. Slice plantains into long oval pieces to desired thickness, about 1/8 1/4 inch thick. Toss in coconut oil and sprinkle with a pinch of sea salt. Place in roasting pan and cover with foil. Cook on low at 320 degrees F for 20 minutes until plantains become soft and slightly puffed up. Remove cover and increase temperature to 420 degrees. Bake for another 15 minutes until lightly brown and crisp on the outside. Serve warm and enjoy.

Jamaican Rice and Gungo Peas

Ingredients:

- 4 cups vegetable stock or water
- 2 lbs. dried gungo peas (pigeon peas)
- 2 lbs. whole grain rice
- 1 stalk scallion
- 1 sprig thyme
- 1 scotch bonnet pepper, whole
- 2 clove garlic, crushed
- 4 pimento berries
- 1 thumb ginger
- 1 cup coconut milk or 2 Tbsp creamed coconut
- 1 tsp sea salt

Directions: Add 2 cups vegetable stock, gungo peas, garlic, pimento and ginger to a large cast-iron pot, cover over high heat and bring to a boil. When gungo peas rise to the top, add 1 cup vegetable stock to sink the peas and let cook until partially tender. Add the scallion, thyme, whole scotch bonnet pepper and cook for 20 minutes until gungo peas are soft and water is reduced to about 1 cup. Lower the heat and add coconut milk (or the creamed coconut with 1 cup water), sea salt, and adjust seasonings to taste. Let simmer for 2 minutes to allow flavors to meld. Add whole-grain rice, stir and turn the flame up high. Cover and allow to come to a boil, then lower to medium flame and allow to steam for 30-40 minutes or until rice grains are tender. Turn the flame low when the water is dried out of the rice. If rice grains are not thoroughly cooked, add a tiny amount of water to the rice and continue steaming until rice is thoroughly cooked. Remove from heat and serve with your main vegetable dish.

Smoked Collard Greens

Ingredients:

- ½ yellow onion sliced
- 3 cloves garlic, minced
- 3 cups vegetable broth
- 1 tsp. smoked salt (or liquid smoke)
- 1 tsp. paprika
- ½ tsp. red pepper flakes
- 2 lbs. collard greens, thoroughly washed and dried
- ½ tsp. black pepper, to taste
- ¼ tsp. cayenne pepper, to taste
- 1-2 Tbsp. grapeseed oil

Directions: Add 1-2 Tbsp. to large deep pot over medium heat. Add onions and garlic, sauté until fragrant and tender. Add in vegetable broth, smoked salt, red pepper flakes, paprika, cayenne and black pepper. Taste and adjust spices to your liking. Reduce heat and bring to a simmer. Add the collard greens and let simmer for 1 hour to 1 ½ hour. Do not boil.   Cooking time may vary. Check greens after 30-45 minutes and cook until greens are dark in color and tender. Serve warm.

Vegan Lasagna

Inspired by Keyana Nikaamen

Ingredients:

- 4 oz fresh spinach
- 1 large eggplant, cut length-wise in 1/2" steaks
- 1 package of seitan-based vegan Italian sausages, crumbled [may substitute with 2 cups of fresh mushrooms, diced]
- 1/2 onion, chopped
- 1 medium red, yellow and orange bell pepper, chopped
- 2 Tbsp of grapeseed oil
- 1/2 tsp oregano
- 1/2 tsp basil
- 1 clove garlic, crushed or 1 teaspoon of minced garlic
- 1 tsp salt
- 1 tsp black pepper
- 2 jars of marinara pasta sauce
- 9-12 lasagna pieces
- 2 packages of vegan mozzarella cheese
- 1 recipe of Cashew Ricotta (see recipe below)

Directions: Prepare 1 recipe of Cashew Ricotta Cheese (below) and set aside. Preheat oven to 350 degrees. Boil lasagna noodles according to package directions; then drain. Heat grapeseed oil in a pan, then add eggplant steaks. Season with salt and pepper. Sauté for 2-3 minutes on each side. Remove from pan and set aside.

Heat grapeseed oil in a pan and add the bell peppers, onions and garlic. Sauté for 2 minutes, then add seitan sausage. Season with salt, pepper, basil and oregano and let cook for 4-5 minutes, stirring occasionally. Add 1 jar marinara sauce, mix together, and let simmer for 1-2 minutes before turning off flame.

In a 9x13 lasagna pan, place a small amount of marinara sauce on the bottom and spread evenly. Place 3 lasagna sheets on top of sauce, covering the bottom of the pan. Layer in this way: cashew ricotta on pasta, followed by sauce, followed by fresh spinach, followed by eggplant, followed by seitan sausage, followed by mozzarella cheese. REPEAT until all is layered. Finish by spreading a thin layer of marina sauce on the last layer of pasta and sprinkle mozzarella on top. Cover with aluminum foil and bake in a preheated oven for 55 minutes. Remove foil and bake for another 15 minutes until cheese is melted. Let sit 10 minutes before serving.

Cashew Ricotta Cheese

Ingredients:

- 1 cup raw cashews, soaked for 2-4 hours (or boiled for 20 minutes until tender)
- 1/2 cup water
- juice of 1 large lemon
- 1 – 2 tablespoons nutritional yeast, optional
- dash of onion powder
- salt cracked pepper, to taste
- 1 teaspoon of oregano and basil

Drain cashews and place all remaining ingredients into a blender (or food processor). Mix well until creamy, stopping to scrape down the sides every few minutes. Taste for flavor, adding any additional ingredients. Season to taste!

Scoop mixture back into an airtight container and place in the refrigerator for up to an hour. This will stiffen the mixture a bit and make it more "ricotta-like." You can also prepare your dish straight away without refrigeration if needed. However, refrigeration will improve the consistency. Enjoy!

References

Note: Afrakan Names are written in correct order, from an Afrakan-centered perspective, to maintain their proper meaning and spiritual energy.

Aqiyl Aniys. *Alkaline Herbal Medicine.* Natural Life Energy LLC., 2016.

Akua Gray. *Natural Health and Wellness Consultant Manual.* BJK Publishing, 2016.

Becker, Robert O., and Selden, Gary. *The Body Electric.* William Morrow and Company, 1985.

Bettelheim, Frederick A., Brown, William, H., and March, Jerry. *Introduction to General Organic, and Biochemistry.* Books/Cole- Thompson Learning, 2004.

Dewald, Jonathan. *Europe 1450 to 1789: Encyclopedia of the Early Modern World.* Charles Scribner & Sons, 2003. 6 vols.

Dudek, Susan G. *Nutrition Essentials for Nursing Practice.* 2001. Lippincott Williams & Wilkins, 1987.

Elsie Nene Obed. *Simple African Recipes.* Conprel Nigeria Limited & Lillies International Inc, n.d.

Gale Cengage Learning. *The Gale Encyclopedia of Diets: A Guide to Health and Nutrition.* Gale Cengage Learning, 2007. 2 vols.

Gardiner, Sir Alan. *Egyptian Grammar.* 2012. Griffith Institute, Ashmolean Museum, Oxford, 1927.

Kats, Solomon, H., and Weaver, William Woys. *Encyclopedia of Food and Culture.* Charles Scribner & Sons, 2002.

Ife Kilamanjaro. Tdka Kilimajaro, & Yahra Aaneb. *African Time Expanded Edition.* University of Kmt Press, 2020.

Llaila O. Afrika. *African Holistic Health.* 2004. World Inc., 1983.

Llaila O. Afrika. *Dictionary of Vitamins and Minerals from A to Z.* Seaburn Publishing Group, 2010.

MacMillan Publishers Limited (2015). "Fat, fibre and cancer risk in African Americans and rural Africans." https://www.nature.com/articles/ncomms7342. *Nature Communications*, Accessed 6 September 2016.

Marshall Cavendish Corporation. *The World and its Peoples: India and its Neighbors Part 1.* Marshall Cavendish Corporation, 2008.

Muata Ashby. *Kemetic Diet.* 2002. Sema Institute of Yoga, 2000 / Cruzian Mustic Books.

Mfundishi Jhutymys Ka N Heru Hassan K. Salim. *The Spiritual Warriors are Healers.* 2016. Charles Child Publishing, 2003.

Nutrition and Well-being A to Z, edited by Delores C.S. James. MacMillan Library Reference, 2004.

Ody, Penelope. *The Complete Medicinal Herbal.* Dorling Kindersley Limited, 1993.

Peirce, Penney. *Frequency: The Power of Personal Vibration.* 2011. First Atria Books, 2009.

Price, Weston A. *Nutrition and Physical Degeneration.* 2008. Price-Pottenger Nutrition Foundation, 1939.

Queen Afua. *The City of Wellness.* African World Books, 2008.

Queen Afua. *Sacred Woman.* The Random House Publishing Group, 2000.

Rekhit Kajara Nia Yaa Nebthet. *RaSekhi Kemetic Reiki Level One.* 2014. Ra Sekhi Arts Temple, 2012.

Rekhit Kajara Nia Yaa Nebthet. *RaSekhi Kemetic Reiki Level Two.* Ra Sekhi Arts Temple, 2013.

Ra Sekhi Arts Temple. *Recipes for Elevation.* Ra Sekhi Arts Temple, 2013.

Sertima, Ivan Van. *They Came Before Columbus.* Random House Trade, 2003.

Sherwood, Keith. *Chakra Therapy*. 2015. Llewllyn Publications, 1988.

Other Works by this author

Mdw Ntchr Flash Cards Volume 1: Alphabet by BaNAuset KaNSekhmet

Mdw Ntchr Flash Cards Volume 2: Biliterals by BaNAuset KaNSekhmet and Basui-mshu Nikaamen

Mdw Ntchr Flash Cards Volume 3: Triliterals by BaNAuset KaNSekhmet and Basui-mshu Nikaamen

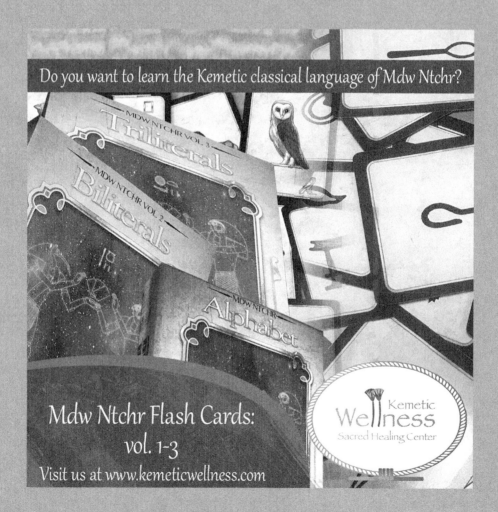

Index

A

B

grand rising chia porridge, 117

grape wine, 61

gratitude, 76, 83

Great Rift Valley, 54

green banana porridge, 131

green bananas, 133-134

grilled jerk eggplant steaks, 139

guacamole, 127

H

halal style, 55

HAty [haty], 103

healing tools, 75, 79

    emotional, 82

    physical, 85

    spiritual, 76

healthy internal environment, 3, 44, 84

healthy skin, 19, 113

heart disease, 51, 65

    prevention, 113

heartburn, 11

heka / hekau, 93

hemophilia, 113

herbal teas, 10, 49, 73

herbal therapy, 88

hieroglyphs, 93

high fructose corn syrup, 38

high protein greens, 9

high vibration foods, 3, 48, 51

high vibration nutrition alternatives, 43

Hinduism, 60, 77

histidine (his), 30

homeostasis, 44

honey nut oats, 118

hoosh, 69

hormone balance, 12

hormone-free, 40

hormones, growth hormones, 40

Horn of Africa, 55

hot breakfast couscous, 136

hot pepper gazpacho, 127

hummus, 11, 61

hydration, 49, 113

hydrogen, 14

hypotension, 26

I

immune system, 5, 14, 24, 33, 85, 113

immune system, 5, 85

    boosts, 14, 24, 33, 113

    dysfunction, 24

    regulation, 15

    weakened, 28

improves cognitive function, 12

Printed in Great Britain
by Amazon